CONTENTIOUS COLLABORATIONS AND SOCIETAL SHIFTS

CONTENTIOUS COLLABORATIONS AND SOCIETAL SHIFTS

a snapshot of the current worlds of healthcare, technology, and business

Justin DeCleene MBA, MIS, PBMCT, CPhT

ISBN: 1547085959
ISBN 13: 9781547085958

Disclaimer

This material is provided for informational purposes only and should not be construed as primary source information. Readers should consult a subject matter expert for specific applications of the content provided herein. Although care has been taken in preparing this material and presenting it accurately, the author and publisher disclaim any express or implied warranty as to the accuracy of any material contained herein and any liability with respect to it. Similarly, although the author has exhaustively researched all sources to ensure the accuracy and completeness of the information contained in this book, the author and publisher assume no responsibility for errors, inaccuracies, omissions, or any other inconsistency herein. Again, although the author has made every effort to provide accurate Internet addresses at the time of publication, neither the publisher nor the author assumes any responsibility for errors or for changes that occur after publication. Further, the author and publisher have no control over, and do not assume any responsibility for, third-party websites or their content. Any attacks against people or organizations are unintentional.

The Silent Rank

I wear no uniform, no Navy blue, or Army green.
But I am in the service, in the ranks rarely seen.
I have no rank upon my shoulders, salutes I do not give.
But the Military work, is the place where I live.

I'm not the one who fires the weapons, nor puts my life on the line.
But my job is just as tough, I'm the one that's left behind.
My Spouse is a Patriot, a brave and prideful man.
And the call to SERVE his country – not all can understand.

Behind the lines I see, the things I needed, to keep this country FREE.
My spouse makes the sacrifice, but so do our kids and me.
I love the person I married; "sailoring" is his life.
But I stand among the silent ranks, known only as a navy wife

Betty DeCleene (1933-2010)

What Life Is All About

Life isn't about keeping score. It's not about how many friends you have. Or how many people call you. Or how accepted or unaccepted you are. Not about if you have plans this weekend. Or if you're alone. It isn't about who you're dating, who you used to date, how many people you've dated, or if you haven't been with anyone at all. It isn't about who you have kissed. It's not about sex. It isn't about who your family is or how much money they have. Or what kind of car you drive. Or where you're sent to school.

It's not about how beautiful or ugly you are. Or what clothes you wear, what shoes you have on, or what kind of music you listen to. It's not about if your hair is blonde, red, black, brown, or green. Or if your skin is too light or too dark.

It's not about what grades you get, how smart you are, how smart everyone else thinks you are, or how smart standardized tests say you are. Or if this teacher likes you, or if this guy/girl likes you. Or what clubs you're in, or how good you are at "your" sport. It's not about representing your whole being on a piece of paper and seeing who will "accept the written you".

But life is about who you love and who you hurt. It's about who you make happy or unhappy purposefully. It's about keeping or betraying trust. It's about friendship, used as sanctity, or as a weapon. It's about what you say and mean, maybe hurtful, maybe heartening. About starting rumors and contributing to petty gossip. It's about what judgments you pass and why. And who your judgments are spread to.

It's about who you've ignored with full control and intention. It's about jealousy, fear, pain, ignorance, and revenge. It's about carrying inner hate and love, letting it grow and spreading it.

But most of all, it's about using your life to touch or poison other people's hearts in such a way that could have never occurred alone. Only you choose the way these hearts are affected and those choices are What Life Is All About.

- Author Unknown

Table of Contents

Justin DeCleene MBA, MIS, PBMCT, CPhT

"We're just getting started on our goal of connecting everyone." That's the goal of Facebook's founder, Mark Zuckerberg. I share that vision. Information should not be something that only privileged students or wealthy people have access to. It should be provided to everyone whether it's in the form of electronic devices or printed material, social media or newspapers, everyone should have access to the same information no matter who they are or where they are.

I am worried about the millions of growing children that do not have access to information. I am worried about their future means of supporting themselves and being contributing members of society. I fear for the dying arts and bodies of knowledge due to a lack of interest in the next generation. That is why I am seeking to inspire the next generation to utilize the vast bodies of information that are available at their fingertips and experience the positive impact it can have on their life. Critics may say that information comes and goes over time, and this is true; however, whatever the duration of availability, whatever the size, a piece of information can have extreme importance and the potential to cause a movement.

I have a dream that the exiting generation will have a positive recollection of the impact they made on the world. I have a dream that the next generation will look back and be amazed at the progress the previous generation made. And lastly, I have a dream that the world experiences an unconscious spreading of knowledge where everyone has equal access and everyone understands it. When I say "generation", I mean any human being living within a given time regardless of race, color, national or ethnic origin, ancestry, age, religion, disability, sex, gender, gender identity, sexual orientation, military, genetic information, or any other characteristic. Feelings around the current state of the world need to be emotions of happiness, pride, and accomplishment. Emotions of anxiety and urgency should be nonexistent.

Here are some of the ways that increasing the access to information can benefit an individual:

1. Increased awareness of the world we live in and subsequent wisdom about why things are the way they are
2. Creative solutions to world problems due to understanding the root cause and history of things

3. A feeling of contentment and decrease in anxiety due to a general lack of the unknown
4. A sense of control and empowerment in one's situation and environment
5. Comfort in lifestyle due to a high position in the workplace
6. Being viewed as a subject matter expert and confidence that colleagues look up to you
7. Improved understanding of various cultures around the world and an appreciation for diversity
8. An increase in empathy for people in various life situations
9. Positively contribute to society, find meaning in life, and adapt to change better

My goal is to paint an unbiased, millennial view of the current world in which we live. There are so many complexities and corners in the fields of Healthcare, Technology, and Business that need to be captured in the literature - all in one place, all in one source. Once this foundation of knowledge is compiled and reviewed, it is then easier for an individual to maintain an ongoing desire of learning.

The Healthcare section applies traditional and contemporary leadership methods to pharmacy practices in retail and institutional settings, explores the collusion of large pharmaceutical companies, and proposes solutions to the currently flawed healthcare system in America. The cost of drugs, the opioid epidemic, and the complexity of the current healthcare system are topics that are examined. The Healthcare section concludes with a piece on technology in healthcare and the difficulty of adoption.

This leads to the Technology section which reviews innovation of the day such as artificial intelligence, cognitive science, internet of things, and privacy. The role of automation, the rise of robots, and the outsourcing of information technology cause debates to ensue. The prominent, conflicting sides are surveyed.

The Business section transitions technology innovation into the realm of business. Technology companies like Microsoft, IBM, Apple, and Google have interesting experiences and diverse philosophies on how their businesses thrive and how they are to operate. This section concludes with a piece on frivolous lawsuits and captures people's sense of entitlement at the time.

I've included a special chapter called "Big, Idealistic Systems" to explore a number of solutions to the current healthcare system's demise. There are numerous proposed solutions to the systemic problem, but they're not being entertained fast enough by the key decision makers. Anyone can be a part of any kind of positive change. It is my hope that the generations to come will leave the world in a better place than when they entered it. There are a multitude of diverse issues, but it only takes one person to initiate the needed solution that can change the world.

How to Read this Book

This book is really two books in one: a book that provides information relevant to the time, and a book that synthesizes and applies the information to the future. The provision of the information provides a framework, and the application provides practical examples for the future. If someone were to learn lots of information, spend half of their life in school, and earn lots of degrees but never apply it - What good is it? I agree that learning for the sake of learning is fine – but there's so much more to experience when information and knowledge are applied to real-life scenarios.

Because of this, I recommend reading this book from start to finish. Understandably, some readers will want to race to the punchline first; however, the punchline is much more meaningful when the foundation is strong. The book can be read for either the application or the background knowledge. But the background knowledge will lead to a better understanding of the application. Again, the first part of each section (Healthcare, Technology, and Business) provides a foundational survey of the knowledge in the field and the second part of each section provides the application of the information.

For your convenience, there are appendices in the back of this book that contain definitions, cited references, and suggested readings so that you can look up, verify, and expanding your knowledge respectively. The seeking of knowledge is continuous. That's why I encourage you to specifically consult the glossary and suggested readings for more information.

Introduction

"When you feel like quitting: Think about why you started."

— Unknown

I still keep in close contact with my best friend from elementary school. We grew up downhill skiing, making bike ramps, and goofing around in school together. We try to video chat at least four times a year to update each other on what has been going on in our lives. The last chat we had started like they usually do: my update on my job and travels and his update on school and his next steps in life. Halfway through the conversation, the tone changed from casual updates to the uncertainty of the future.

We both started questioning the point of higher education, what we wanted from life, how we were going to pay our student loans, and how we were going to achieve everything we wanted to. Most millennials like me are asking these same questions. There are lots of uncertainties in America's healthcare system and economy. This causes grave concern on how people will support themselves and thrive amidst struggles, broken systems, and lots of unknowns. I am anxious and excited about the future of innovation, but at the same time, I'm scared and concerned for how my generation will support itself and what legacy it will leave behind. We all have a responsibility to potentiate the spread of information and general societal change. This is why I wrote this book. With information, comes power.

This is no shortcut to obtain vast amounts of information about the current world in which we live. There is no substitute to reading newspapers, magazines, academic journals, and online articles. I advocate for the old-fashioned reading of printed materials in order to obtain primary source information. It may seem to others like you are naturally smart, or a genius, or that you catch on quickly. None of that is accomplished overnight. It takes time, dedication, interest, and motivation.

Again, my goal is show you how to single-handedly obtain, consume, and synthesize knowledge that is reliable, informative, and useful.

I'm elated about the notion of obtaining knowledge, digesting it, and spreading it around. Are you excited? Do you wish to be the owner of your own destiny? Would you rather struggle through life, going from paycheck to paycheck, or would you rather have comfort and peace in the knowledge that encompasses the world? Questions that lead to restlessness, anxiety, and urgency may keep you up at night like:

"Will I leave a meaningful, lasting legacy?"
"Will I be happy while I'm on Earth?"
"Will I spend my last days having no regrets?"
"Will I not have to go through the motions for the rest of my life?"

If you are like most people, you wish you can say yes to all those questions... but you can't.

> *Education is what remains after one has forgotten what one has learned in school.*
>
> — ALBERT EINSTEIN (1879–1955)

If you are worried that you're alone and isolated on this journey to knowledge and self-actualization, know that you are not. This is a common feeling. There are humps to get over, but it can be done. This book serves as a diving board into the soaking bath of information. There are methods, secrets, and advancements in the fields of healthcare, technology, and business that are examined in this book. This book serves to inform the reader, and apply the information to real world scenarios.

This book shows you the benefits and techniques of consuming information to improve one's awareness of the current world. The goal is to be self-sufficient in obtaining knowledge, determining facts from falsehoods, and creating an opinion for yourself.

This book references a number of appendices that are located in the back of this book for your convenience. Appendix A is a glossary of the abbreviations that are used in this book along with their definitions. Appendix B contains the cited and uncited references in this book. Appendix C is a list of recommended reading for anyone interested in learning more about the philosophical or practical implications of today.

I wrote this book based on the knowledge and experience I've gained as a student and a worker in the healthcare, technology, and business arenas. I am not a doctor, chief information officer, or a head of a company. I have earned a Master's in Business Administration (MBA), a Masters in Information Science (MIS), a Bachelor's in Science of Chemistry, and I hold many pharmacy technician certifications and licenses at the state and national levels. However, the best advisors are specialists. I work in many areas in my job, but I am a generalist. This allows me to consult others and gain insight into targeted solutions so I can weigh the pros and cons, make an informed decision, troubleshoot, and further consult members of my team.

As a final disclaimer, the methods I share in this book are for purposes of surveying only. For example, I am not in favor of one method of leadership over another. I'm just examining the most popular avenues in hope that the reader will form their own opinion of them and create their own, strong justification of why they are in favor of that path.

The video chat encounter that I shared with you at the top of this section illustrates the need for and the reason why I wrote this book. My goal is to inspire people and spread information. I sincerely hope that people will become lifelong learners. I imagine that video chats, or whatever means of communication, in the future will be more positive and effectuate change in a better direction. I have faith in my generation. I have hope for my generation. We all have a role in the world we live in. Hopefully, upon the exit of my generation, we will have left the world a better place than when we found it. Decades from now I hope that the generation of the time will look back at my generation and appreciate the progress that has been made and the positive, accepting, and sustainable environment that exists. The time for change is right now and an unconscious spreading of knowledge where everyone has access and everyone understands it can aid in this world improvement venture.

> *"The facts of the present won't sit still for a portrait. They are constantly vibrating, full of clutter, and confusion."*

> – WILLIAM MACNEILE DIXON,
> PROFESSOR OF LITERATURE

The Current State

The early 21st century in America was a time of health, economic, political, and safety struggles. This period in America filled many history books, many sport records were beat, advances were made, but also a serious period of economic hardship was present. Stressing over the economy, people turned to eating and shopping which made many people gain weight and become bankrupt. Having pre-existing health conditions would prevent people from obtaining health insurance. Some people needed food stamps from the government to buy food. People were diagnosed with, survived, and died from cancer.

People loved shopping. Most people ended up shopping outside of their means. Credit card bills grew and credit scores dropped. This made banks think twice before lending money to customers. Once people realized they could not afford things, people made efforts to save money. They started staying at home, cooking healthy dinners, and cutting back on shopping. Since people were not buying as much as they used to, there was less of a demand for products, which decreased the need for jobs. Companies were cutting back hours, wages, and laying people off. Many American citizens were out of work. This caused an increase of competition among applicants in the job market.

Children came from many backgrounds and races. Some were more fortunate than others: parents got along, went on several trips, and had a second home. Others were constantly surrounded in conflicts at home. There were bomb threats written in bathroom stalls of middle schools and students picking up trash in the hallway. While some skateboard the streets looking for approval, others wrote books. There were students that could not afford to eat at school, and others that went on ski trips without their parents.

Many students were under pressures that they created for themselves: trying to look like models, worrying about the flawlessness of their skin, or how fit they were. This caused many teens to feel worthless and depressed when they didn't meet these standards. To temporarily relieve their depression and feelings of isolation, teens cut themselves, smoked, drank, or played dangerous games like the gasping game. Some teens did these things till they took their own life. Where were the parents? They were either too busy working to provide a childhood for their kids or they were struggling with an addiction.

With not being able to afford necessities, some children turned to a life of crime to get what they needed. The teen prostitution rate noticeably grew. The average age was 13. The younger generation was longing for acceptance. Many of their fathers were absent. They did things with other teens and older men to feel accepted and to fill a void their parents left. They viewed selling their body as a quick way to get cash for the designer clothes they wanted. Lastly, teens wore more expensive apparel (ie: ninety dollar shoes, fifty dollar shirts, etc.) and were more open to talking about private issues.

Global Warming was also a big topic of discussion. Some people thought Global Warming was caused by CO_2 omissions, while others thought it was part of the Earth's natural cycle. Polar ice caps began shrinking causing a 0.7°C difference in temperature each year. When ice melts, it leaves water. This water got left in the oceans and lead to the rising of shorelines. If the government did not act quickly, a lot would be at stake:

You see that pale, blue dot? That's us. Everything that has ever happened in all of human history, has happened on that pixel. All the triumphs and all the tragedies, all the wars, all the famines, all the major advances... it's our only home. And that is what is at stake, our ability to live on planet Earth, to have a future as a civilization. (Guggenheim, 2006)

We needed to protect that civilization. We needed to protect our home. The early 21st century was a time of many emotions and triumphs. It was a time of many successes and failures.

COEXISTING GENERATIONS

Four generations coexisted in the 21st century. This explained the highly diverse, fragmented markets that were present. The Baby Boomers (born 1946 to 1964) controlled 70% of US disposable income. They bought two-thirds of the new cars, half the new computers, and a third of the movie theater tickets on the market annually. They spent about $105 a day in 2015. The next generation was born 1965-1982. They were known as Generation X and were all grown up with teenage kids. They heavily cared for their older parents and splurged rarely on themselves.

Within Generation X is a subset of people known as DINKs (Double Income, No Kids). Raising a kid born in 2013 cost $245,000-340,000. That's a lot of extra money! This subgroup had second homes, expensive hobbies, and took lavish vacations. The final generation was the Millennials (born 1982 to 2004). Jobs went south just as they were entering the job market. Millennials were health-conscious, married to technology, and owners of college debt. They also preferred to spend money on experiences (ie: vacations) rather than material possessions. The generations could be cross-classified by their social and financial status. Some of the richest people in America were known as the One Percenters. They were unaffected by the Great Recession of '08. This group's consumption consisted of luxurious cars and yachts, million dollar watches, and passion purchases on items like rare art pieces.

POLITICS

Politics were a large part of this period in America. There were numerous debates and arguments where candidates placed blame on each other. Presidents did what they thought was best for their country (ie: going to war with terrorists; fixing economic, health, and climate issues, etc.). Due to the strongly divided political climate of the twenty-first century, and impart due to Facebook, a social movement was born.

"The Other 98%" was a national movement that stood up against the strong influence that big organizations and lobbyists had on the United States' democracy. The group felt that as long as corporations had such influence in the American Political System, the change that Americans wanted would never happen ("The Other 98% - About", 2010). "The Other 98%" movement was not the only group that advocated for The People; there were a few groups that fought for the idea that our democracy and the economy should serve the everyday American, not the elite CEOs and lobbyists.

"The Other 99%" movement came one year after the inception of "The Other 98%" ("The Other 98%", 2017). "The Other 99%" is a movement that sprung from updated economical estimates that stated the richest 1% of America had as much wealth as the rest of all America. The group rallied for women's rights, drug price reduction, and the taxing of wealth rather than consumption ("Oxfam says wealth of richest 1%", 2016). The group's poem greatly captured their goals and perspective:

Who are we? Well, who are you? If you're reading this, there's a 99 percent chance that you're one of us.

You're someone who doesn't know whether there's going to be enough money to make this month's rent.
You're someone who gets sick and toughs it out because you'll never afford the hospital bills.
You're someone who's trying to move a mountain of debt that never seems to get any smaller no matter how hard you try.

You do all the things you're supposed to do.
You buy store brands. You get a second job.
You take classes to improve your skills.
But it's not enough. It's never enough.

The anxiety, the frustration, the powerlessness is still there, hovering like a storm crow.

Every month you make it is a victory, but a Pyrrhic one – once you're over the hump, all you can do is think about the next one and how much harder it's all going to be.

They say it's because you're lazy. They say it's because you make poor choices.
They say it's because you're spoiled. If you'd only apply yourself a little more, worked a little harder, planned a little better, things would go well for you. Why do you need more help? Haven't they helped you enough?
They say you have no one to blame but yourself. They say it's all your fault.

They are the 1 percent. They are the banks, the mortgage industry, the insurance industry.
They are the important ones. They need help and get bailed out and are praised as job creators.
We need help and get nothing and are called entitled.
We live in a society made for them, not for us.
It's their world, not ours. If we're lucky, they'll let us work in it so long as we don't question the extent of their charity.

We are the 99 percent.
We are everyone else. And we will no longer be silent.
It's time the 1 percent got to know us a little better.

("We Are the 99 Percent", 2017)

ADULTING

Adults in the twenty-first century severely struggled with work-life balance. This was such a struggle that it was given the name "adulting" (ie: "I'm having a hard time adulating."). Some struggles of work-life balance include managing personal relationships, family, and work demands. Adulting can be especially difficult if one is on shiftwork. Shiftwork is when an employee's hours of work rotate between daylight and nighttime hours. Studies have shown that shiftwork leads to obesity, a high consumption of junk food, early aging, and a lack of sleep ("I'll Sleep When I'm Dead", 2016). Ultimately, it is certain that adulting can be circumvented by adopting a few lifestyle changes.

A few changes to one's daily routine can greatly impact how one copes with adulting. A lack of motivation is a common condition among adults. Employers also have a huge role in this. Ways of wasting time at work can result in lots of motivation (Greenfield, 2015). If employers offer times throughout the workday for things like free meals, massages, and even animal shelter fundraisers, employees' productivity increases. Similarly, if something makes one feel good, he/she will do more of it. If something makes one feel horrible, maybe one should back off a little (Brodesser-Akner, 2016).

NO MEANS NOTHING

The 21st century was an era that experienced a complex shift in society's attitudes toward sexual assault towards woman. There are two pieces of mainstream media that greatly contributed to this shift: the television series Law and Order: Special Victims Unit (SVU) and the book series "Fifty Shades of Grey" by E. L. James. There was one episode of SVU that demonstrates this shift in thinking, incorporates the Fifty Shades book series, and the impact (both good and bad) that the books have had on society's attitudes towards sexual assault towards women.

On season 14 episode 3 of SVU, a character named Jocelyn Paley wrote a book called "Twenty-Five Acts". The book, like "Fifty Shades of Grey", revolutionized women's attitudes about sex. On the surface, it was a book about sexual fantasies, desire, and kink. In reality, it was an empowering erotic novel about women getting what *they* want. Jocelyn appeared on a talk show called "Raising Cain" to promote her book. She greets him with a quick, flirtatious kiss. After the show, Cain and Jocelyn go out for a fancy, romantic dinner. She coyly removes her underwear and hands them to Cain under the dinner table.

Later in the evening, they go to Cain's apartment and get intimate. As he starts to remove his belt, he says, "Act two. I say when you can touch me" (Zimmer, 2012). He orders her to get on all fours and whips her with his belt. She says that really hurt and tells him to stop. He responds by choking her hard with the belt. She gasps as he whispers, "You don't tell me what to do!" The next morning, Jocelyn reports the rape encounter to Manhattan's Special Victims Unit. Initially Jocelyn is hesitant to even call it a rape because she flirted with Cain all night and told him to dominate her. Detective Amanda Rollins asks Sargent Benson if she read Jocelyn's book. Rollins informs her of Act 5 where the protagonist was choked with a belt and had eighteen orgasms. The following night, there was a party where Cain toasted to Jocelyn. She was freaked out and started to leave. Cain chases her into the elevator. He is furious that she went to the cops. Cain hikes up her skirt and sodomizes her again. The detectives at SVU watched the security tape and noted that it didn't look like Jocelyn resisted (Zimmer, 2012). Benson and Rollins state there are three possible responses of a victim: fight, flight, and freeze.

Tonic immobility, freezing, is a phenomenon where someone under stress panics and can't move. Assistant District Attorney (ADA) Raphael Barba meets with Rollins and Benson and asks them if Jocelyn seems credible. He asks because a recent jury on a strangulation case read Jocelyn's book and failed to render a verdict. ADA Barba meets with Jocelyn and warns her that the one thing in her personal history that she leaves out is the one thing the defense will use against her to win the case. Back at the squad, the other detectives did some research on Cain and found that Cain tends to prey on young girls new to the city. Rollins found that Cain prematurely leaked his monologue and Cain warns that he's going to be falsely accused of raping author Jocelyn Paley. Detective Nick Amaro comments that it was a smart move for Cain to get in front of the accusation. Benson is concerned that Cain can use his talk show as a bully pulpit. Benson and Rollins speak to a former employee of Cain and she reports that he's a good guy until he gets the belt in his hands, then he loses it.

Under cross examination, the defense attacks Jocelyn by revealing that Jocelyn is not the actual author, but that the author is an English professor by the name of Kathleen Dobson. The jury made the correct and swift decision to convict Cain. Even if this wasn't the result, the victim typically is empowered by confronting their assailant. With all that Jocelyn endured, despite the fact that she said "No", it's natural for one to ponder the social norm of having a "safe word". If Jocelyn had a "safe word", would it have prevented her assault? If Jocelyn would have been less flirtatious, would it have prevented her assault? These are typical questions that arise when blaming the victim (Leotta, 2012). It shouldn't matter. No means no. No should mean something. Although there's been improvement in prosecuting and punishing sexual assaults, there's still more work to be done to ensure victim blaming is put to rest.

CREATIVE DRUGS AND THE GAP BETWEEN LAW AND HEALTH

Kratom is a green leaf of a tree of the coffee family. It's been used for centuries in Indonesia, Malaysia, and Thailand. The leaf has been gaining popularity in the US, but not for the original use of boosting energy. Taking 2-3 grams of Kratom is said to induce euphoria and reduce pain while not experiencing the side effects of prescription opioids (Gruley, 2016). This is all great news: an alternative pain relieving agent that is an unregulated plant. Initial data from the University of Florida shows the demographic with the highest usage is white, employed and educated males between 31 and 50 years old with a salary of at least $75,000 per year.

Despite the benefits of Kratom, the Food and Drug Administration (FDA) and the Drug Enforcement Agency (DEA) are working to classify the plant as Schedule I which would prevent the promising studies and treatments from ever coming to fruition. Contrary to the positive case studies of patients using Kratom, the DEA and FDA have seen some patients enduring negative side effects from Kratom (Gruley, 2016). Patients getting sick, going through withdrawals upon stopping treatment, and the illegal smuggling of the substance across national borders highly tempts American regulatory bodies to classify Kratom as a Schedule I drug. Whether it's bath salts, Kratom, or the latest trending drug, the regulatory bodies will always be playing catchup.

CONCLUSION

The 21st century was an interesting time in America's history. The generation of the time was faced with lots of uncertainties. It was a pivotal point in time where the future could either be drastically improved or rapidly decay further. The economic, healthcare, and political systems were inefficient and unsustainable for the current and future generations. There was an urgent need for thought leaders and innovators to make a difference. It took a while for the system to get this broken; it will take even longer to get it back on track. Severe pressure to improve the world is on the shoulders of Millennials. We need to leave the world better than when we entered. We need to leave a meaningful legacy behind. I believe that the spreading of information is the first step to these hefty endeavors.

Book 1: Pharmacy Management and Leadership

2

Leadership Application: Healthcare

"Give me a lever long enough and a ful-crum on which to place it and I shall move the world."

- ARCHIMEDES

INTRODUCTION

"I would prefer to spend time discussing briefly our greatest need in hospital pharmacy – leadership" (Francke, 1955). The need to discuss pharmacy leadership is still relevant today. There is a great lack of leadership that still exists in the pharmacy profession. Leadership comprises capacity, goals, and efficacy. Hospital organizations are unique because they are comprised of many diverse units that work together for a common goal. Each of those units need strong leaders to guide their staff to achieve clinical outcomes. The pharmacy department is no exception.

THEORETICAL FRAMEWORK
There are only a few accredited pharmacy management or leadership residencies. Sara White, a distinguished resident of the American Society of Health-System Pharmacists (ASHP), believes there are seven elements of leadership:

1. Have a written work group vision and mission.
2. Work effectively to accomplish actual results.
3. Persevere and persist.
4. Influence through attitude and approach.
5. Work well with others.
6. Lead oneself so people want to work with the leader.
7. Invest in the future.

(2006)

These elements revolve around better employees, the organization, and of course, the patient. Succinctly, White puts it, "Leaders are disciplined, patient, assertive, confident, and accountable" (2006, p. 1498). There are many attributes that good leaders have and these should be incorporated into specific leadership training for the pharmacy profession.

Hospital pharmacy is a very complex department within a medical system. There are many subsections within a pharmacy department which makes it difficult for the pharmacy manager. Generically speaking, systems thinking is especially relevant to the pharmacy department (Scahill, 2008). In order for the manager to know whether or not policies are working, he/she must think about how all of the subdivisions work together. The manager needs to find out if and where there is a gap in the system and find the best way to fix it. The ASHP published an audit about hospital pharmacy services. Reflecting upon the audit, Higby (2014) noticed reoccurring patterns and themes in great hospital pharmacy services. He constructed "leadership lessons" that should be applied to these services to make them more beneficial, not only to patients, but also to the employees that work in the department. The top lessons are: obtain outside help and expertise as needed; analyze, digest, and think; and have clear objectives (Higby, 2014). Leaders should integrate knowledge from multiple sources in order to make the best decisions.

Good leadership starts at the hiring process. Organizations need employees that independently lead but also follow their managers. In order for managers to hire leader-worthy employees, the hiring process should be reexamined, modified, and improved (O'Connor, 2013). O'Connor (2013) says that "process change comes from the bottom-up, but culture change moves from the top-down" (p. 391). It may take time, but a pharmacy manager should lead the process of implementing a new and stricter pre-employment screening process.

As previously discussed, the hiring process should be modified to select applicants with great leadership skills and experiences. That is difficult to do if there are few people that have those skills. In 2005, Sara White distributed a survey on pharmacy leadership. The survey revealed that 34% of pharmacists are less satisfied than they were five years ago. It also showed that 44% of pharmacists are planning on continuing in their practice for 5-10 years; additionally, 26% said they will retire after they leave their position (White, 2005). This shows that there will be a large surge in the need for pharmacists with leadership skills. In another one of White's articles, she concludes with a great, applicable piece of advice. She states, "If you question why things are a certain way and you are not satisfied with 'that's the way we've always done it,' then forge a new path with answers that are more satisfactory" (White, 2006, p. 1503). Great leaders have intrinsic motivation to question policies and critically change things if necessary.

APPLICATION

Retail Pharmacy

Pharmacies are high stress workplaces. Retail settings are even more stressful. At a retail pharmacy that I worked in, I had a manager who controlled his emotions and empathized with customers and employees. When an angry customer came in, he worked with them calmly and figured out what they needed or what the breakdown in communication was. He didn't let his emotions cloud his focus, judgment, or tone. His impulses were minimized and controlled. When working with his coworkers, he changed his tone to appeal to each one on an individual basis. He exercised emotional intelligence. He talked to his staff pharmacist with a professional tone of instruction and management. When he talked to the lead technician he empathized with all of the pressure she was under and all the tasks she had to complete. When he talked to me he kept it concise and mostly work-related because he could tell my personality did not welcome off-subject chatter. Lastly, he talked to interns like a friend and tried to make them feel welcomed, but at the same time, provided them with great educational opportunities.

Hospital Pharmacy

At a hospital pharmacy that I worked in, the director seemed like she had no stress. She didn't acknowledge any of the many issues present in the organization. She went on as if everything was fine and functional. She looked over people's shoulders to see if they were working. She was very concerned with policies and whether or not the employees were following them even if they're not in the best interest of the patient. She was naïve and had no concept of the realities that occurred in the pharmacy department.

The supervisor at the hospital added stress to her workers. She was not nice and went around adding duties and changing policies without approval from anyone else. One day she made two workers cry. The workers got so worked up because she wanted them to do something different that was not even something they could control. In another instance, she entered the pharmacy yelling at the top of her lungs because the staff they did not read her latest email she sent an hour ago with a policy change. The policy would be something like putting medication boxes on one counter versus another. In the end, that does not have implications on patient safety. If the boxes are stocked by technicians and checked and signed off by pharmacists, there is no issue in the system; therefore, the manager should not have focused her attention on a policy like that since it doesn't fix anything.

She was the reason for the discord and anxiety that ran rampant in the organization. There was no sense of pride or leadership. Everyone was for themselves and passed blame onto each other. The management should have shown more empathy and motivation to increase worker's morale and ultimately employ emotional intelligence. She should have thought critically before she implemented new policies. This would have increased adherence among employees because confusion around the changing policies would decrease.

CALL TO ACTION

Since PharmDs are not trained in leadership, it is important to have someone study pharmacy leadership that is trained in business and has pharmacy experience. There are some accredited pharmacy residencies that teach leadership and management, but many students do not have access to them. Sara White (2006), a distinguished American Society of Health-System Pharmacists (ASHP) resident, believes there are seven elements of leadership, a few of them include: influencing through attitude and approach; working effectively to accomplish actual results; and leading oneself so people want to work with the leader. Succinctly, White puts it, "Leaders are disciplined, patient, assertive, confident, and accountable" (White, 2006, p. 1498). There are many attributes that good leaders have. With the known lack of leadership training in the pharmacy profession, there needs to be an industry-wide change.

There needs to be a shift in focus from vision and mission statements, expectations, and policies to trusting employees more to use their abilities and training. Clark agrees with Granko when he says, "trust is an essential element of leaders and managers" (Clark, Kokko, & White, 2012; Granko, Morton, & Schaafsma, 2013). Patients trust pharmacists for accurate prescription information. There not only needs to be trust between pharmacists and their patients, but also between managers and their workers. Trust is an important component of the leadership definition. Wu, Yang, & Chiang (2012) believe that "leadership may act as a catalyst for trust, communication, and shared values" (p. 714). Effective leadership allows trust between the manager and his/her employees which results in better employee productivity and ultimately better clinical outcomes. In order to combat the lack of leadership professionals in the upcoming years, there needs to be mentoring programs in place. The issue with mentorship programs is that they add stress to current professionals that already have numerous demands on their schedule (O'Connor, 2013). A good leader and pharmacy manager would allow pharmacists to lighten their workloads in order to train the leaders of tomorrow.

CONCLUSION

Trust allows managers to let their employees lead and share their ideas which can create success and innovation. Organizations that have a trusting and diverse culture have an advantage in recruiting and retaining employees (Clark et al, 2012). Leadership allows for an environment where thoughts can be openly communicated at all times.

A pharmacy department is very complex and vital to any medical institution. There are numerous sub-processes and employees within the pharmacy department which makes it difficult for the pharmacy manager to do his/her job. In order for the manager to know if policies are working, he/she must think about how all of the subdivisions work together. The manager needs to find out if and where there is a break in the system.

A high degree of planning and coordination is exhibited by good leaders. It is common in the healthcare setting to have leadership teams. Some teams may have five different professionals. Each of them are from different disciplines in order to provide the patient with the most treatment options and best knowledge possible. Galli and Handley (2014) described shared leadership in teams as "leadership that is created when individual members influence other members" (2004). Leaders can usually make any changes they want, but in the end, it matters how the changes are perceived and followed by the employees. Everyone on a team should be able to lead and represent their own point of view.

3

Organizational Structure in Hospital Pharmacies

The Healthcare sector is rather dynamic and complex. It is a conglomerate of prescribers, pharmacists, nurses, emergency services, surgery, insurance companies, contracts, IT data management, automation, robotics, rehabilitation, and the list goes on. Somehow there is continuity between all of these segments; however, the communication between the segments usually suffers. In order for any company to thrive in this industry, it's important that the main focus is on the patients. Patient communication is key and will be the main differentiating factor for healthcare institutions. It is also important that patients fully understand their rights and why they are provided the services that they are provided. A collaborative environment coupled with ample business experience can be beneficial for both patients and organizations.

Seddon suggests that managers ditch the traditional top-down hierarchy. An approach that they should follow is the "think system": where people's performance is governed by the system in which they work. A hospital pharmacy strives to identify errors and the parts of the system that causes the errors. Doing that alone is not enough as they also need to implement the change that is necessary to prevent those errors in the future.

BOGSAT

A "bunch of guys sitting around and talking". This is not just a common occurrence in everyday life; this is an important business phenomenon. It is not enough for leaders to act as cogs in a machine; they need to perform a valuable, useful service that benefits the organization as a whole. Reed, the director of Command and Leadership Studies at the United States Army War College in Carlisle and the person that coined the term "BOGSAT", reiterates that systems are created by people; therefore, systems can fail if not maintained properly (2006). This regularly happens in the field of pharmacy when numerous committees, with good intentions, try to identify problems, but they fail to rectify the issues by implementing the necessary change. Reed also identified a common issue of many managers, where their own urgency displaces importance. Many pressures are placed on managers by multiple functional areas; these stressors often negatively affect management. The stressors take precedent over the immediate change that needs to happen in order to maintain basic daily operations.

Senge believes that organizations should not focus on making mistakes (1990). At the pharmacy, everything is date, time, and name stamped. If anyone makes a mistake, they were called out in a meeting by upper management and asked to identify what went wrong. This was good because it identifies the mistake, but at the same time, it shames the person that made the mistake. This does not make people feel comfortable and it does not foster a learning environment. This correlates with Senge's concept of "the top leads and the local act". Employees need to feel like they are a part of an organization. They need to feel like their thoughts count and that their talents are utilized appropriately. Pharmacies and other healthcare settings typically have a culture where the practitioner "knows all".

OPERATIONAL STATISTICS

Ackoff believes the goal of an organization's subdivision needs to be looked at from the prescriptive from the whole organization. Management often acknowledged how fast the medications need to reach the nurse, but failed to pay attention to the time that it takes for the nurse to administer the medication. The ultimate goal is for the nurse to administer the medication on-time according to the doctor's orders. Many steps go into that: the pharmacy needs to produce, verify, and deliver the medications on-time, and then the nurse needs to receive the medication in order to administer the medication to the patient on-time. The nurses have many patients to manage; therefore, by the time to medication reaches them, they may be busy with another patient. The pharmacy failed to account for these extra times when looking at the operational statistics when evaluating the performance of the employees within the pharmacy.

One Organizational Process

A patient wants to fill a drug at a pharmacy that was pre-scribed by their doctor. However, this drug is not on the insurance's formulary; therefore, a prior authorization is required. A prior authorization is a complex process that involves communication between the insurance company, the prescriber, the patient, and the pharmacy. It is rather difficult to receive, track, and document communications between these parties. Now multiply this by 5,000 and that's the average volume of what insurance companies deal with every month in regards to prior authorizations. This is just one complex process that usually has to com-ply with certain federal laws. Patient appeal rights can also complicate these organizational processes. The good news is that steps can be taken to improve these processes.

ORGANIZATIONAL MODELS

Theory

The business unit approach allows for fewer workers to directly report to the CEO, more cohesion within units, and more accountability. The units have managers that work closely with their workers and manage small groups.

The CEO cannot have decision-making authority in this approach. Company executives work closely together to assess unit profitability (Heynold & Rosander, 2006). The units coordinate and communicate tasks between them. One unit is devoted to shared services such as financials. Other decentralized units such as accounting and budgeting allow for an efficient support structure that is able to meet the needs of all the units. Units should have clearly written agreements on how communication is exchanged between them. This model frees up work hours, allows unit managers to negotiate competitive labor terms, and focus on profitability. The degree of differentiation allows the right amount of accountability and number of connections so that one person does not have too much power.

A mechanistic model is one that has individual specialization, simple integrating mechanisms, centralization, and standardization. An organic model is one that has shared specialization, complex integrating mechanisms, decentralization, and neutral adjustment. The fundamental model is mechanistic and the workers are individually specialized. In a fundamental model workers essentially work alone and there is no collaboration. The model has simple working relationships and departments are centralized to one location.

Application of the Model

The business unit model is organic. There are many complex organizational relationships and inter-workings in the business unit model. Lots of collaboration and team work allow for neutral adjustment. The shared specialization allows for small changes in business without the managers approval, and relies on individual expertise. Many units have the same services decentralized throughout them.

In the hospital that I worked at, there were many departments that worked together to provide safe and effective healthcare to patients. There were decentralized health care professionals throughout the units providing their different services. Pharmacists provided medication management, sonographers provided ultrasounds, lab personnel measured values, nurses provided care, doctors provided diagnoses, and nutritionists provided the most effective meal plan. These units had to abide by protocols and procedures set forth by medical boards. If nurses only acted on professional judgment, there probably would be more medical mistakes than there already are. Protocols are in place to maximize patient safety. All of the units reported to an executive board comprised of VPs and presidents of other units and business departments. This executive board usually reports to the President of the hospital.

In short, the inpatient hospital pharmacy looked at the parts before it looked at the whole. According to Ackoff, they should look at the whole first, and then the parts. This would help them determine how the parts would operate. So in terms of the pharmacy analyzing their process, they succeeded at taking the system apart and understanding what each piece did, but they fail to understand what the parts do for the whole.

CONCLUSION

A hospital can be considered both mechanistic and organic. It is mechanistic in the clinical sense that healthcare workers need to abide by set protocols and report to a board. It is organic because they do not directly report to a CEO, they collaborate between units, have set ways of doing so, and there are decentralized roles. Most importantly, healthcare is constantly changing. Rare diseases emerge, new medications are discovered; therefore, a large amount of decisions are left to "professional judgment".

4

The Goal

*"Sometimes, it's about the small victories –
if you want to think big, don't be afraid to
start small."*

— ANDREW BATTLEY

Companies are comprised of various divisions in order to not only produce something or provide a service, but to accomplish a common goal. This goal needs to be clear and there needs to be ways to measure the progress in achieving the goal. A novel by Eliyahu Goldratt, entitled *The Goal*, provides ways to measure and maintain the goal of an organization (Goldratt & Cox, 2012). Throughput, inventory, and operating expenses are just three measures that are useful when monitoring the progress of a company's goal.

Throughput is the rate that valuable output is generated by sales. Inventory is the money invested in the products to be sold. Lastly, operating expense is the money that allows inventory to become final products. Keeping throughput up, inventory down, and operating expense down does not necessarily mean the business will be achieving its goal. The goal always needs to be monitored against itself, ie: gains in profit, not just "profit." Throughput, inventory, and operating expenses are ways to evaluate the goal of a business.

Goldratt has a five-step process, known as the Theory of Constraints, to help a business reach their goal of increasing profit. The process is based on increasing throughput. First, before the process even begins, the business needs to identify the goal of the company: to make money. The first step is to find the bottleneck. Bottlenecks are resources where the demand is greater than the ability or capacity of that resource. Then, all of the bottleneck decisions need to be made the highest priority. If the bottleneck still cannot keep up, resources such as people and machines should be added to support the bottleneck and increase its throughput. The last step is to evaluate, re-evaluate, and maintain the system. By the end of this process, the goal should still be valid, and if it is not, step one needs to be revisited.

Pharmacies are a growing business. It seems like there is a retail pharmacy on every corner. Pharmacies hold a lot of liability. There are many steps and policies involved

in order to provide safe medications to the communities they serve. Pharmacies in hospitals have different processes that are followed when dispensing medications to patients. A hospital pharmacy is responsible for verifying and filling orders, tracking inventory, providing patient counseling, obtaining medications at the best price, and supplying all of the units with narcotics and emergency medications. Much staffing, training, documenting, and monitoring is needed to run an inpatient pharmacy.

A pharmacist's job is to provide safe medications to patients for the purpose of bettering their health. Inventory, in this context, is medications. Throughput is the rate at which medications are verified, filled, and dispensed. Throughput is dependent on sales, or in this case, the number of prescriptions. This is ultimately dependent upon the population of the hospital, or general community population. There are many operational expenses: water, power, staff wages, office supplies, medical supplies, and technology.

Goldratt's process can be applied to pharmacy. There are many processes involved in dispensing medications; therefore, there are many places for bottlenecks to exist. Each process is dependent upon the type of medication. For simplicity, the dispensing of an insulin pen in a hospital pharmacy will be considered. The steps are as follows:

1. Doctor submits the order for the insulin pen.
2. Pharmacist verifies the order and prints the label.

3. Pharmacy technician gets the insulin pen from the fridge, writes a 28 day expiration date on the pen, labels the pen, scans two barcodes, and signs the label.
4. Pharmacist verifies the completed order.
5. Technician hand delivers the insulin pen to the medication room on the unit.

The first step in the Theory of Constraints is to find the bottleneck. In this case, a bottleneck could be a machine or a staff member. The dispensing of an insulin pen does not involve any machines because insulin cannot be stored in any dispensing robot and it is not able to be tubed, or electronically delivered, to the unit. Possible staff bottlenecks include the doctor, the technician, and the pharmacist. Since the doctor is outside the pharmacy and is an uncontrollable precursor to the process, that staff position will not be considered as a possible bottleneck in this setting and process

Two possible places for bottlenecks remain: the pharmacist and the technician. When the pharmacy is busy during the day, pharmacists need to verify dosing, check dispensing machines, check IV and oral syringes, answer phones, and collaborate with doctors, nurses, and technicians. Technicians need to answer phones, tube or hand deliver medications, fill orders, stock medication bins and shelves, compound IV bags, set-up and restock dispensing robots, and collaborate with pharmacists and nurses.

In conclusion, pharmacists are the bottleneck. The pharmacist, and not the technician, is the bottleneck for one reason: there are always more technicians than pharmacists working in any pharmacy. Since the bottleneck is determined, it needs to run constantly. One way of making sure this happens is to have another pharmacist. Prioritizing orders is usually already in effect. Certain medication bags are labeled "STAT" or "WAITING" to indicate that the administration time is approaching and the medication needs to reach the patient faster than the other "routine" medication orders.

The third step is to make the bottleneck of utmost importance. To implement this, if the pharmacist needs anything changed or grabbed from another location in the pharmacy, a technician should stop what they are doing and help the pharmacist. If this change still leaves the pharmacist unable to complete his/her job in a timely manner, two options remain. The first option is to have a less busy pharmacist help the hot seat during peak times. Peak times are when doctors are on patient rounds in the morning and are submitting many new orders. The second option is to staff two hot seat pharmacists during the day to get the job done and satisfy the goal.

Preferably, from a business standpoint, option one would be enough to complete the job. If not, option two would come at a higher cost, but it may be necessary to ensure patient safety and timely throughput. If the goal isn't reached, more expenses could arise due to malpractice lawsuits or compliance violations. The final step is to evaluate the bottleneck and to make sure the ultimate goal is still being pursued. The author of *The Goal*, Eliyahu Goldratt, conjured up an idea known as the Theory of Constraints. This five step process is a tool that businesses can implement in order to reach their ultimate goal. This process is applicable across many types of business disciplines. The Theory of Constraints is a way to help businesses increase productivity, profit, and make their overall more efficient.

5

Performance Appraisal Systems

DUTIES AND RESPONSIBILITIES OF A CERTIFIED PHARMACY TECHNICIAN

Pharmacy Technicians are responsible for filling medication orders efficiently and accurately. They compound intravenous (IV) medications, antibiotic creams, and label individual doses of tablets, capsules, and liquid formulations. Simply put they do anything to assist the pharmacists. Pharmacy Technicians, whether in a hospital or community setting, serve under the direct supervision of the pharmacist. Some skills that are required for pharmacy technicians are basic knowledge of the metric system, types of pharmaceutical dosage forms, and drug nomenclature. Other necessary skills are the ability to do ratio calculations and retrieve and enter orders from prescribers.

SELF-ASSESSMENTS

Some characteristics of a good pharmacy technician are preferring to work on many tasks at once, scheduling more things than they can handle, guilty feelings during periods of relaxation time, and impatience with things that occur slowly. These are all characteristics of a type A person. Type A people seem to succeed in the healthcare industry. Another assessment that provides a good picture of what it means to be a good pharmacy technician is a personality test. Motives are things that drive people to behave a certain way. They explain why people do what they do. A good pharmacy technician is a natural goal setter, sees the whole picture, and is highly disciplined. People who are motivated by power and are driven to succeed make good pharmacy technicians.

A final assessment that is applicable to the pharmacy technician position is the ethical decision making skills test. This test is comprised of 50 scenarios and the testtaker needs to select the best action to take in the given scenario. Ethical decisions are important in this position because technicians are constantly faced with different actions they could take, and it's up to them to remain ethical and follow established guidelines. If there is no precedent in the scenario, then the employee needs to use their best ethical judgment and be able to back up their decision if they are questioned later by upper-management.

BACKGROUND ON PERFORMANCE APPRAISAL SYSTEMS

Due to the diverse ways to structure of organizations, there are many different approaches to create the most effective performance appraisal system. Some common types of appraisal systems are building up, breaking down, weakness-based, and strength-based (Aguinis, Gottfredson, & Joo, 2012a). No matter which appraisal system is implemented, there are five concepts that need to be evaluated: relevance, sensitivity, reliability, acceptability, and practicality (Cascio, 1982). With these variables in mind, it is no surprise that most appraisal systems are ineffective. Most of the time, managers are not trained to properly conduct effective appraisal interviews. There is a lack of accountability, and a lack of incentives provided to the managers to supervise their workers effectively (Cascio, 2011). It is difficult for everyone involved because no one system works for all positions or companies. As Scott and Einstein (2001) say, one size does not fit all. This causes appraisal systems to be difficult to manage.

Fortunately there are ways to predict which appraisal system will work better than others in a given organizational structure. However, there is no clear-cut way to pick the best system. There are common shortcomings in many appraisal systems. There are documented ways to rectify them. Biases and the lack of training of assessor's are common shortcomings of appraisal systems. Some solutions for these shortcomings include setting goals for what performance appraisals need to accomplish, focusing on behavior and results, and improving the performance appraisal process in order to increase manager compliance with completing them (Kondrasuk, 2012). There are many options to obtain the ideal system for a particular position.

CURRENT STATE

Multi-source Feedback (MSF) is a common practice in appraisal systems today. Specifically, a Mini Peer Assessment Tool (Mini-PAT) has been studied and tested in a hospital to see how doctors, nurses, and pharmacists rate junior pharmacists and other pharmacy staff. The results showed that doctors and nurses rated pharmacy staff higher than their pharmacy co-workers (Patel, Sharma, West, Bates, Davies, & Abdel-Tawab, 2011). The efficacy of an appraisal system is strongly correlated with who is doing the appraisal. The system's reliability needs to be tested. Patel et al (2011) rendered Multi-source Feedback useless. The feedback is only helpful when the supervisor is conducting the appraisal. The assessor needs to observe the assessee's work first-hand and be familiar with their performance (Aguinis, Joo, & Gottfredson, 2012b). Multiple, inexperienced assessors lead to ineffective feedback.

A survey was done in community pharmacies to determine if technicians are receiving useful feedback, if any. Desselle, Vaughan, & Faria (2002) provided a list of job functions and responsibilities to technicians and pharmacists. The participants of the study were told to rank the functions according to importance. The pharmacists and technicians ranked the responsibilities the same. The study showed that the technicians want more formal feedback, but there was not a proper system in place to provide technicians with "workable feedback" (Desselle et al, 2002). The authors suggested that actions be taken to implement a system that is behavioral-based so that organizational demands can be met and technicians know how to improve their performance.

RECOMMENDATIONS

Performance appraisal systems usually utilize some free-text comments. This is an area for supervisors to write down anything they think the employees can improve upon or praise them for their great achievements. Vivekananda-Schmidt, MacKillop, Crossley, & Wade (2013) found that in the clinical setting, free-text feedback comments are not effective in improving the employee's personal development and performance. It was observed that there was a major disconnect between the comments made by the assessors and those made by the assessee. The assessor's comments were not centered on the assessee's personal development, but rather on what characteristics the assessor thought were important. Free-text feedback comments proved to be ineffective and should not be used for pharmacy technician performance appraisals in clinical settings.

As mentioned previously, performance appraisals vary widely and certain ones are only successful in a given setting. Some of the things that have to be taken into consideration are that systems need to be behavioral-based and the person doing the assessment should be trained. The only person that should be assessing the technician is the lead technician, the one who is in contact with the assessee the most. Even if lots of changes to the system are made, assessors may still not be reviewing properly (Farndale & Kelliher, 2013). A factor in effective performance appraisal systems that is not thought of too frequently is culture. It is important for employees to identify issues in the appraisal system that are related to cultural differences. The more that culture is integrated positively into performance appraisals, the lower the employee turnover rate and absenteeism will be (Peretz & Fried, 2012). The more accurate the performance appraisal, the more the company will benefit due to having effective employees.

It is important that the appraisal system be behavior-based because there is much teamwork involved in the job. Good employees help their co-workers out whenever possible and they work as a team to get the job done accurately and efficiently. Also, the system needs to be implemented with assessors who are trained properly. Perhaps, there should be a practical component of the appraisal if the assessor has not been able to closely monitor the employee. The employee could be told to compound a certain medication and could be assessed on the technique and cleanliness of their work.

Another thing that could make an appraisal system effective in the pharmacy setting is having the assessor providing work-able feedback. That is, giving the employee something that they can work on and have the progress tracked. Goals should be set and monitored for the employees. If they are not meeting the goals, further coaching should be done. However, the appraisal system should not become a negative thing (Aguinis, Joo, & Gottfredson, 2011). The assessor needs to remain understanding and show empathy to the employee.

Key Performance Indicators (KPIs) are sometimes reviewed by managers in order to assess the behavior and performance of employees. Some examples of KPIs that pharmacy technician supervisors may look at are time to fill a prescription, percentage of prescriptions filled correctly, and the number of surveys with positive feedback that mention a specific employee. KPIs do not always have to be related to employee performance. They can also be related to costs, customer satisfaction, and the safety of the business (Ishaq Bhatti, Awam, Razaq, 2013). Only KPIs that the employee has direct control of should factor into employee appraisals. Typically managers rely heavily on these, but in an effective performance appraisal system, KPIs are just one part of the picture that completes the employee's overall performance assessment.

CONCLUSION

Performance appraisals are usually viewed negatively by employees. This is because assessors usually focus on giving negative feedback and not positive feedback (Aguinis et al, 2011). In order to combat this, Aguinis et al (2012a) suggests that for every negative comment, the assessor should give three positive comments. Having the appraisals done in a positive manner will cause the manager to give a better appraisal and the employee to better utilize the feedback. In conclusion, there are many approaches in creating effective appraisal systems. There are many ways to approach modifying a performance appraisal system in order to meet the needs of the company. Managers need to be trained to give effective appraisals, the assessor needs to have witnessed the assessee's performance, and the feedback needs to be specific and accurate (Aguinis et al, 2012). As Scott and Einstein (2001) would agree with me, there is a critical need for the implementation of effective appraisal systems and there are steps to take in order to accomplish such a task.

6

Training Methods and Their Effectiveness

The pharmacy field is constantly changing and is a career that is currently in high demand. More pharmacy schools are being built and hold the responsibility of training the pharmacists of the future. Due to accreditation standards set by the Accreditation Council for Pharmacy Education (ACPE), programs are expected to have their students complete Introductory Pharmacy Practice Experiences (IPPEs) and Advanced Pharmacy Practice Experiences (APPEs). ACPE sets little requirements for these programs; therefore, much discretion is left to the school. IPPEs and APPEs are the only on-site training pharmacists are required to do in any PharmD program. Pharmacists may also do an optional residency program after they complete the PharmD program.

There are various models of training that schools employ: simulations, rotations (IPPEs and APPEs), and residencies. There has been some research done as to what methods of teaching allow students to learn most effectively. In general, simulations are becoming more prevalent in the education arena. Whether they are physical or virtual simulations, studies show they are equally beneficial to students. Typically schools have students do 8-five week rotations to satisfy the APPE requirement. However, a pharmacy school in Florida has their students complete all of the APPEs at the same institution. There are advantages and disadvantages to this model.

Lastly, pharmacy residencies overall are being revised. With much advancement in pharmaceuticals, residencies are expanding in time and content. Some suggest that residencies should be extended from two years to three years to be able to include more training on leadership skills. Others suggest APPEs should have more rigid criteria in place for accreditation purposes. The proposed revisions of pharmaceutical residencies have been compared to that of a medical residency. Some models of training are more effective than others for preparing pharmacists for certain situations in a clinical setting. Health fields are rapidly advancing. Because of this, people being trained in these fields need to be trained at a higher level than previous students. Pharmacy is one of the fields in the healthcare sector that needs to reevaluate how schools are training their upcoming professionals. Schools utilize simulations and optional residencies to give their students more hands-on experience. Certain training models are more effective than others in producing clinical pharmacists.

SIMULATIONS

Simulations are a cheap, effective way to give students hands-on experience at an early stage in their pharmacy education. There are many types of simulations: high-fidelity patient models, standardized patients, virtual reality, and full environment simulations (Lin, 2011). Research has shown that no matter what kind of simulation is used, students' learning is improved. ACPE does recognize simulations as a way to teach critical thinking and problem-solving skills (Mieure, 2010). There have been publications speculating that IPPEs may be replaced by simulations since many things learned in IPPE can be learned through simulations. Simulations are a way to replicate real-life scenarios that students encounter in a clinical setting.

Pharmacy schools have the responsibility of teaching their students many skills. The specific skills may cause one type of simulation to be more effective than another. For instance, if an instructor is trying to teach students how to measure blood pressure, the instructors should use a programmable computerized patient simulator rather than a human subject (Seybert, 2007). This is because blood pressure changes constantly; therefore, if a patient is used, it's hard for the instructor to verify if the student's reading is correct. Human patient simulators are people acting to be like other healthcare professionals, patients, or patient's family members. The University of Alabama at Birmingham uses human patient simulations to teach their students how to professionally interact in a clinical setting.

They created a room devoted to housing the simulation. An instructor at the university explained, "We observed the pharmacy students interact in a genuine, caring, and professional ways" (Tofil, 2010, p. 4). There are many uses for simulators in pharmacy education.

No matter how advanced simulations are, nothing can replace the real environment. Advantages to training with simulations include that there is no risk to live patients, no preceptor is necessary, and the ability to repeatedly practice. Disadvantages include the fact that a simulation is not a real scenario, human emotions and personalities are absent, and costs may be high (Lin, 2011). An important observation is that sometimes effectiveness of a simulation increases when group discussions and lectures simultaneously complement the simulation (Benedict, 2010). It is important that the appropriate simulation is selected, advantages and disadvantages are considered, and if possible, lecture content coincides with the simulation.

IPPE AND APPE ROTATIONS

IPPEs and APPEs are another tool that schools use to make sure their students are prepared for their future careers. Young, Vos, Cantrell, & Shaw (2014) and a team of pharmacists did a study on what students thought made an excellent preceptor. The study had students complete a fourteen item evaluation on their preceptor. The scientists realized that "ACPE provides minimal oversight on how preceptors should be evaluated by students" (Young et al,

2014, p. 3). Because of the lack of criteria, the pharmacy school is left with much discretion in regards to what their APPEs contain and how to improve them. Lastly, Young and his team found that students preferred preceptors with skills in "serving as a role model, showing an interest in teaching, and relating to the student as an individual" (2014, p. 5). Students did not care about the pharmacist's certification, degree, or years of experience.

Some pharmacy schools are taking the initiative to improve their APPEs even though they are not required to by ACPE. Hatton and Weitzel published an article on how converting the traditional 8-five week rotation APPE model to a block schedule system affected their student's learning at the University of Florida College of Pharmacy (UFCOP). First they tried to formulate what an ideal APPE model would look like: "[it] would provide students with many opportunities for learning, incentivize preceptors and institutions, and ensure high-quality educational experiences" (Hatton & Weitzel, 2013, p. 2145). The authors believed that the block schedule decreased logistical arrangements of traveling to multiple rotation sites, allowed more time for students to develop skills, and formed more relationships with students and staff. Students would help each other through the rotation, provide Warfarin and discharge counseling, and learn more in-depth concepts. Patient satisfaction increased and the hospital became recognized both regionally and nationally for the projects their students worked on.

There are noted disadvantages to the block schedule system: students only get to experience one institution, technology is hard to provide to that many students while on rounds, and near the end of the APPE, students get comfortable and essentially become free labor to the institution (Hatton & Weitzel, 2013). Another way to improve APPEs was discussed at the end of Young's article. He suggested that preceptors should be required to complete "training on how to serve as a role model, make time for students, and provide good direction and feedback" (Young et al., 2014, p. 5). The block schedule and preceptor training are just a couple of ways to improve the APPEs.

A pharmacy school in Vancouver tested an APPE model that placed students in a long term care (LTC) facility where their preceptor was off-site. Usually the doctors and pharmacists that work at LTC facilities rotate between multiple LTC sites. The rotation put a student at one LTC facility and the preceptor rotated between sites. This approach is called "role-emergent" compared to the "role-established" model. The study showed that the LTC staff "felt that they delivered better care to residents as a result of the services provided by the students" (Kassam, Kwong, & Collins, 2013, p. 9). Preceptors also said they learned new skills from the students. As a result of the role-emergent model for APPEs, students, preceptors, site staff, and patients were benefited. The authors hope these findings will cause LTC facilities to be viewed as rotation sites that offer "legitimate institutional-based learning experiences"

(Kassam et al., 2013, p. 10). The role-emergent model allows students to take ownership and have a great deal of responsibility for the professional duties they conduct in the LTC facilities.

RESIDENCIES

Residency, or post-graduate training, is a way to gain additional clinical experience. Residencies are typically two years and there are not many residency positions available, despite the high demand. In addition to the few positions open, a lack of funding, coupled with the fact that these opportunities are not presented to students until their third or fourth year of pharmacy school are some reasons why students forgo residencies (McCarthy & Weber, 2013; Clark, 2014). Scholars weigh many options like costs and value when deciding to pursue post-graduate training (Hagemeir & Murawski, 2014). Many think that a residency is a prerequisite for a pharmacy job in a hospital, but that is not true (McCarthy & Weber, 2013).

A lack of funding and lack of residency programs are the biggest issues with pharmacy training today. Johnson and Teeters did research on the current state of pharmacy schools with regards to quality. They identified areas that needed improvement, and how these improvements should be implemented. They explained the current state of the pharmacy profession as, "similar to the [problems] the medical profession navigated through fifty years ago" (Johnson & Teeters, 2011, p. 1546). There are a few ways to combat the issues. Johnson suggests that in order to increase funding, someone must document what takes place during a residency, how patient satisfaction increases, and how the hospital benefits.

Clark and Johnson have some ideas on how to improve the current residency model too. Clark thinks that adding another year, PGY3, will allow graduates to learn how to succeed in a leadership role within a hospital. Pharmacists are becoming integrated with other hospital staff such as doctors, nurses, and lab personnel. Johnson believes that having the current post-graduates teach the incoming post-graduates will allow a more efficient flow of graduates in and out of residencies. This way the pharmacy director of the institution will not have to train so many students and this will allow more residency opportunities. Perhaps a quicker way of opening up residency positions is to create non-hospital residencies, such as community pharmacy residencies.

CONCLUSION

Training is a critical part of any business. It is directly related to the success of the business. Pharmacist training begins in school. Learning clinical applications and techniques is a major part of what pharmacy school teaches. Simulations, IPPEs and APPEs, and residencies are ways for students to build their clinical expertise inside and outside of pharmacy school. Rotations and residencies are being improved to meet the needs of students as the world of pharmacy expands. There has been success when multiple types of learning are used together. Neal Benedict, a professor at the University of Pittsburg school of pharmacy, used "computer-assisted learning (CAL), virtual patient technology, branched-outcome decision making, guided group discussion, and lecture" (Benedict, 2010, p. 1). Quality learning takes place when multiple teaching methods are used in synergy. The way pharmacists are trained needs to be continually reevaluated in order to train pharmacists effectively in a dynamic field and prepare them to excel in a professional, clinical setting.

7

A Balanced Scorecard

INTRODUCTION

A balanced scorecard allows for the identification of measures that align with an organization's strategic goals so they can be tracked over time (Rough, McDaniel, & Rinehart, 2010). Pharmacies have to have an extremely high level of quality assurance in order to meet the goals of patient safety and improving patients' health. Currently, there is a severe lack of standardized metrics for pharmacies in general (Livin, Hertig, & Hultgren, 2013; Nau, 2009; Brown, 2009). If one were to look at metrics for chain pharmacies, they would look extremely different than health-system pharmacies. A balanced scorecard analysis reveals that health-system pharmacies must carefully consider the metrics they use in order to achieve their strategic objectives.

THEORETICAL FRAMEWORK

Not much literature has been published on pharmacy metrics and workflow. Livin, Hertig, and Hultgren (2013) found forty-three articles pertaining to Health IT metrics. They noticed thirty-four metrics that varied widely. Health IT metrics can be used to assess employees, workflows, and investments in technology. Primarily, metrics are used to assess and reduce medication errors ("Reduce medication errors", 2009). They can also be used to see how safety is impacted by the processes that are in place (Livin, Hertig, & Hultgren, 2013). The following are suggested metrics for hospital pharmacies that have been published in the literature that deal with benchmarking and productivity:

Suggested Internal Pharmacy Benchmarking Productivity Monitoring Indicators:

- Worked hours per unit of service
- Drug cost per admission
- Labor cost per admission
- Total cost per admission
- Doses dispensed per admission
- Labor expense per 1000 doses billed
- Pharmacist worked hours per order
- Technician worked hours per dose

- Inventory turns per year
- Clinical interventions per pharmacist shift worked
- Pharmacist: technician skill mix ratio
- Pharmacy cost as a percentage of total hospital costs

(Rough, McDaniel, & Rinehart, 2010)

Decentralized clinical pharmacy productivity metrics:

- Orders verified in EMR
- Orders entered into EMR (oral)
- Orders discontinued
- Patient profile review
- Progress notes
- Unexpected medication event reporting
- Emergency resuscitation code attendance
- Clinical Pharmacy Interventions (per month or year)

(Pawloski, Cusick, & Amborn, 2011)

Potential areas of the balanced scorecard include financial health, operational efficiency, customer service, employee satisfaction, external quality standards, and clinical effectiveness (Rough, McDaniel, & Rinehart, 2010). Some metrics used internally are:

Process	Measurement
Product procurement, storage, retrieval, and preparation	Orders placed, line items ordered, purchases percentage on contract, product stock-out rate, shorted items necessitating development of a substitution process, total parenteral nutrient solutions mixed, complex admixtures
Drug distribution	ADC stock-out rate, ADC override rate, ADC actions performed for pharmacy (refills/loads/unloads)
Order management	Orders reviewed (entered) per period, order review (entry) turnaround time
Clinical practice	Clinical documentation rate (interventions per adjusted discharge)
Other quality indicators	Clinical opportunities identified versus performed
Financial outcomes	Drug expenses per statistic
Workload	Work force hours per worked unit of service, ratio of staffed versus filled positions, total 100 workload units

(Rough, McDaniel, & Rinehart, 2010)

The following are examples of productivity ratios that can be used to assess how the staff in the pharmacy department is working:

Examples of Labor Productivity Ratios	Examples of Cost-Based Productivity Ratios
Hours worked per adjusted patient day *(hours worked per 100 CMI-weighted revenue-adjusted patient days, hours worked per 100 pharmacy-intensity score-weighted patient days)*	Drug cost per adjusted patient day
Hours worked per adjusted discharge	Labor cost per adjusted patient day
Hours worked (paid) per 100 orders processed	Total pharmacy cost per adjusted patient day
Hours worked per 100 admissions	Drug cost per adjusted discharge
Hours paid per adjusted patient day	Labor cost per adjusted discharge
Hours paid per adjusted discharge	Total pharmacy cost per adjusted discharge
Hours worked per patient day	Drug cost per 100 orders processed
FTEs per dose billed	Labor cost per 100 orders processed
FTEs per order processed	Total pharmacy cost per 100 orders processed

FTEs per occupied bed
FTEs per adjusted patient day

(Rough, McDaniel, & Rinehart, 2010)

Metrics can be used to measure a variety of things: productivity, processes, financials, satisfaction, and clinical objectives. Due to the multiplicity of metrics, there are varying sources that metrics can originate from. Some sources include: prescription records, administrative claims, operational records, and patient reports (Nau, 2009). Due to the lack of consensus in the literature surrounding metrics in health-systems pharmacy, it is rather difficult to construct a balanced scorecard. However, there are some reoccurring concepts that should be included. Surveys can help collect metrics as well. The Hospital Consumer Assessment of Healthcare Providers and Systems (HCAHPS) Survey collects data on every hospital in the United States that collects reimbursement from Medicare and/or Medicaid. It is a national standard that primarily measures patient satisfaction to allow valid comparisons between hospitals ("Patient survey (HCAHPS)", 2015).

APPLIED THEORY OF BALANCED SCORECARDS

Financials

Financial objectives of a pharmacy are to maintain and secure monetary assets to ensure organizational stability. This is done by maximizing revenue, managing operating costs, and minimizing staff working hours. The minimization of staff working hours helps to manage operating costs. Most of a hospital's revenue comes from the pharmacy department because drugs are expensive. In the end, monitoring the amount of hours that employees work, the costs of drugs, and the amount the hospital charges patients for the drugs will ensure long-term financial stability.

The two biggest costs of the pharmacy department are the cost of drugs and the cost to dispense the drugs. The cost of dispensing drugs includes employee wages and operating costs (ie: technology, electricity, office supplies, etc.). Therefore, some appropriate metrics for this category include drug cost per admission (drug cost without insurance to have a standard pricing scheme because insurance benefits greatly differ), pharmacy operating costs to hospital operating costs ratio each month, working hours per 100 orders processed, and full-time employees (FTEs) per order processed (Rough, McDaniel, & Rinehart, 2010). The last metric alludes to productivity which reflects operating costs. If some employees can get the same amount of work done faster than other employees, then their work should be evaluated in the effort of reducing costs and increasing the financial stability of the pharmacy department.

The organization should minimize costs and carefully examine working hours which indirectly measure cost. Drug costs per admission should be around $20,000 because the majority of patients only need allergy, asthma, and/or antacid agents, while others need chemotherapeutics. Chemotherapy agents can be $20,000 per dose while the other agents can be $1.00 per dose. Therefore these figures balance out. The pharmacy operating cost to hospital operating cost ratio is around 1 in 4 because although drugs are expensive, surgeries, medical supplies, and technology costs add up. The remaining two targets are dependent upon the workload of the particular health-system pharmacy. Financial indicators in the pharmacy department measure the ultimate goal of maintaining financial stability.

Patient

Typically on a balanced scorecard, there is a section for customers. In a hospital setting, the clients or customers are called patients. They are the stakeholders. They chose which hospital they get admitted to and they have the power to improve the hospital just as much as the executive staff does. Patient objectives of the pharmacy include: providing industry leading patient care and identifying improvement opportunities. In order for a hospital to become a leader in their industry, they need to demonstrate service excellence to their patients. After all, they are providing a service to their patients that aim to improve their health.

Measurements of patient care should properly assess how well the patient is being cared for. Appropriate metrics include: the number of patient deaths, readmission rate for the same condition, and HCAHPS Patient survey responses (Pawloski, Cusick, & Amborn, 2011). The readmission rate for the same condition is important because that demonstrates how effective the clinical staff was in treating the condition the first time that the patient came into the hospital. The HCAHPS survey is an important standardized metric of hospitals that measures cleanliness, communication, responsiveness, pain management, discharge information, and care transition ("Patient survey (HCAHPS)", 2015). Therefore it is important to include the survey in the balanced scorecard.

Most of the targets in this category are zero because there is no room for error in regards to patient safety and there is no other option than improving the health of the patient. The HCAHPS survey measures various things about a hospital and it is an important indicator that the general public and insurance companies use. Some questions are in a Likert-like format, others are short answer. Therefore, the targets for the survey vary by question.

In the patient category, an initiative that can be taken is conducting executive round-robin meetings. A campaign to increase the patient survey response rate has also improved patient satisfaction. The daily executive departmental round robin meetings is when a team of five hospital executives goes around to each department of the hospital for ten minutes to discuss the department's issues, progress, needs, and operational metrics. Some metrics include the number of deaths, patients, incidents, and catheter-associated urinary tract infections (CAUTIs). These short meetings raise important points to leadership of the hospital so that necessary change can happen from the top-down to benefit the patient. The campaign to increase the patient survey response rate includes sending emails and hanging posters throughout the hospital to remind patients to take the survey.

Patient Safety

Internal processes within the pharmacy department allow the flow of medications from the outside vendor to the patient. Numerous processes exist in-between the source of the drugs and the dispensing of them. Patient safety should always be the focus of all these processes because that is the end goal. Internal process objectives of the pharmacy include categories of patient safety, knowledge management, Health IT, and Department Service Excellence. Patient Safety involves anything that contributes to the bettering of the patient and not harming them. Correct medications and the oversight of all safety incidents contribute to the bettering of patients.

Patient safety is a measure that needs to be regularly monitored to prevent any incidents from occurring. Some measures of patient safety that are important to include on a balanced scorecard include: percent of correctly dispensed medications, number of incidents, percent of medications packaged correctly. Rough, McDaniel, & Rinehart (2010b) and Pawloski, Cusick, & Amborn (2011) suggest that the pharmacist to technician ratio should also be included. This ratio needs to be in compliance with state laws. The ratio also alludes to patient safety because there should be a certain number of pharmacists present to properly supervise a given number of technicians. Although at face value these measures may not seem to be related to patient safety, if monitored, they can help prevent incidents that cause harm to patients. The percentages should be 100% because they measure accuracy. Number of incidents should be zero because incidents are usually harmful to patients and should be avoided at all times.

Patent safety is at the heart of all operations within a hospital. By having the medications to be dispensed checked more times by different pharmacists, conducting post-incident review meetings, and complying with state and federal laws, the hospital can improve patient safety when dispensing medications. The dispensing of a medication goes through many steps: selecting the drug, labeling, scanning, and verifying. Numerous staff members are involved in these steps. Therefore it is necessary for multiple checks to be in place to ensure accountability and safety. By educating employees about prior safety incidents they can be prevented in the future. Federal and state laws are usually in place to benefit the patient. Complying with the laws can help protect the patient. These three initiatives are vital for patient safety.

Knowledge Management

Knowledge management is concerned with ensuring that all practitioners share their expertise in order to contribute to the safety of the patient. Some objectives include providing effective medicine reconciliation services, having pharmacists on the rounds team, and having pharmacists stationed in the unit. The presence of pharmacists is essential throughout the hospital to ensure that medications are administered properly and for appropriate reasons. Knowledge management can seem like an abstract category because it is an intangible asset, but it is measurable. Some measures of knowledge management are the percent of medical teams that have a pharmacist and the percentage of units that have a pharmacist stationed on the floor. Rough et al (2010b) and Pawloski (2011) suggest that the percentage of patients that receive a clinical intervention from a pharmacist should also be included. Interventions help remove unnecessary medications from a patient's regime and fix incorrect dosages. When knowledge management is properly executed, it can be a powerful tool for ensuring patient safety and teamwork.

All of the targets should be 100% because, ideally, the pharmacists should be completely utilized throughout the hospital.

Medication reconciliation is a very important service provided to the patient by the pharmacy department. It allows pharmacists to share their knowledge about drugs with the patient and to verify that the patient's profile is up-to-date. Pharmacists can adjust dosages and change medications that are therapeutically duplicate or inappropriate. This also leads to improved patient safety. Sometimes hospitals have criteria that patients must meet in order to qualify for this service such as having three or more chronic conditions or being on anticoagulants. Those criteria should be lessened in order to provide the service to more patients. Also, increasing the presence of pharmacists around the hospital in general allows easier access to medication-related questions.

Health IT

Technology is increasingly being introduced to hospitals. Computers store medical records, dispense medications, and even perform surgeries. It is important from an internal process perspective that these technological components are properly managed to keep processes running smooth and ensure that the safety of the patients are at optimal levels. Therefore, the availability, accuracy, usage, and security of these components need to be managed appropriately in an effort to benefit the patient.

Although Health IT is a big, new area in hospitals, there is little research currently done on how to measure and assess such technologies in hospitals. Some metrics include: percent machine downtime, number of technology failures, percent of application usage, and number of unauthorized access. The majority of Health IT metrics should have targets of zero because they relate to downtime, failures, and a lack of security. Hospitals are institutions that need to operate 24 hours a day; therefore, the technology needs to be running 24 hours. When technology has failures, it has major implications for employee productivity, but most importantly, for patient safety. If a barcode scanner goes out, drugs cannot be verified by all of the available methods; therefore, it is pertinent for these targets to be minimal or zero. Although, the usage metric should be 30-80% to demonstrate that the application is needed, it should not be over-used so it does not deplete the system of its resources.

Improving the availability of technology to maintain inventory and patient safety requires vast initiatives from the hospital. Some initiatives could be having an IT pharmacist seated in the pharmacy and attending daily meetings. An IT pharmacist is typically responsible for maintaining all technology in the department. They are a registered pharmacist who can handle controlled substances, compound drugs, and dispense medications. Technology components that the IT pharmacist maintains can be anything from hard drives and printers to automated dispensing machines and barcoding systems. Having an IT pharmacist can greatly improve Health IT within the pharmacy department. Lastly, HIPPA monitoring should be conducted to make sure the systems are secure.

Department Service Excellence

Department service excellence deals with ensuring the staff is professional and knowledgeable, but also that the department is maintained properly. This area includes: keeping inventory low, properly disposing of expiring medications, and dispensing medications according to documented policies and procedures. Motivation to maintain service excellence comes from within. Professionalism is learned, not innate. The department leaders should lead by example and demonstrate to the staff how processes should be carried out. It is not enough for employees to just do a process, they need to have a questioning attitude and interact respectfully with co-workers.

It is rather difficult to measure professionalism; however, there are some numerical metrics that have proven useful. In addition to professionalism, these metrics also monitor productivity and individual contribution to the department's workload. Some of the metrics include: average time to dispense medications, number of internal survey responses, and percent of new published medical facts that are presented at daily meetings. Rough et al (2010b) and Pawloski et al (2011) suggest that the following should also be included: number of orders entered into the EMR per day, orders verified in the EMR per day, annual inventory turns, and number of expired medications in the pharmacy. The number of orders entered and verified in the EMR should be equal and there should be no expired medications in the pharmacy.

This is perhaps the hardest category to implement initiatives. Continual process improvement can lead to beneficial changes for not only employees but also patients. Improving processes can allow patients to get their medications sooner, return to a healthy state faster, and lead to an overall improvement of the hospital's image. The continual aspect of this initiative is important because pharmacy laws and drug information changes often. Managers need to be receptive to constant feedback and critically evaluate it to see if the feedback has merit and should be implemented. Constant feedback can lead to process improvement which benefits everyone.

Some organizations have an internal survey that employees are highly encouraged to complete. The survey usually asks for opinions the employee has of their department, co-workers, supervisors, and overall image of the organization. There can be useful information drawn from the survey. If positive changes are made to the department that originated from the survey, employees will be happier, more productive, and more dedicated to the organization. The lead clinical director is responsible for educating employees on the latest information and implementing the information into the department's everyday activities. By having the pharmacy director present new clinical information at daily meetings, employees will have the latest information and will be better equipped to make sound clinical judgments. This is essential in department service excellence: service the patient by making the best decision with the latest information.

Learning and Growth

Learning and growth aids in the development of employees which leads to more capable employees. Learning and growth objectives of the pharmacy include ensuring the staff's skills are current and accurate. Learning systems, budgets, and assessments can help with developing employees' knowledge in their field. A degree can only train and educate a person to a certain extent. The person needs to go through annual training in order to stay up-to-date on the latest medical information. This is especially important in the medical field. Like knowledge management, at first glance, learning and growth may seem intangible and difficult to measure. Some tangible measures for these objectives include the number of outstanding learning modules, number of employees that fail the annual injection assessment, percentage of expired certifications and licenses, and percentage of employees that received training within the year. In order to ensure the staff's skills and knowledge, all of the metrics should be zero. These measures have targets of zero because they are framed in a way that reflects poorly on employees. Staff failing assessments, not completing learning modules, and expired certifications are not positive things. For the benefit of the organization, these metrics should be as close to zero as possible. When these metrics are zero, it demonstrates to management that the staff is up-to-date with their training, education, and certification requirements.

Organizations need to set the advancement of their employees as a high priority. Organizations can update employee learning systems, mandate annual injection technique assessments, implement a new application to store employee credential information, and setup a budget for employee training. Updating the employee learning application can allow supervisors to closely monitor which employees have not completed their modules. It also can allow for new modules to be easily added. The annual injection technique assessment ensures that employees have the proper skills to compound IV drugs. An improper technique can cause contamination of the medication. Any employee that fails the assessment has to undergo a week of training by a supervisor until they can pass the assessment. The creation of a new budget for training allows more pharmacists to complete their continuing education credits (CEs) and even travel to some conferences for professional development.

CONCLUSION
Balanced scorecards allow management to assess the state of their organization. They can cause improvement within

the organization to allow for the best possible treatment of the patients. Despite the lack of research surrounding balanced scorecards within health-system pharmacies, there are measurements and initiatives that can be implemented to improve the pharmacy department. Balanced scorecards in the current literature are not individualized to a specific type of organization. Most seem to forget that balanced scorecard components change based on the type of organization. Some important components that should be included, but are often overlooked, are patient safety, knowledge management, and Health IT. Because of the hospital setting, most metrics are either zero or 100 percent. Many situations in the hospital are either life or death; therefore, it is critical to have an effective balanced scorecard in place.

Book 2:
Big Pharma

8

Big Agenda

"You have brains in your head, you have feet in your shoes; you can steer yourself in any direction you choose."

– Dr. Seuss

Big Pharma, the name we collectively attach to all of the drug companies, has been under scrutiny for the past few decades. The government, healthcare institutions, and drug companies collaborate together to supposedly provide us with the finest drugs for our consumption to maintain or improve our health. Peter Coy puts it perfectly, Big Pharma subscribes to a "Machiavellian, long-running, high-stakes Game of Thrones involving: drug makers, insurance companies, pharmacies, PBMs, congress, and presidential candidates" (Coy, 2016). If someone was to simply create a new system, it'd involve the untangling of rebates, reimbursements, pass-through, copayments, and fees. The main concern of the drug companies is not the welfare of the patient, rather, it is how much money they are making or losing.

Almost half of all Americans take at least one prescription drug. Odds are that someone or someone they know has had issues with insurance covering their medications or issues relating to prescriptions not working as intended. Sometimes drugs are sold for the wrong reason and new side effects are not discovered until the patient dies, becomes a paraplegic, or has severe organ damage. Some drugs are not doing what they are prescribed to do because of the dishonesty and bribery among companies. From over-the-counter to prescription to illegal drugs, drugs are a big part of our world. In the end, everyone is affected by drugs. It is important that articles in mainstream media uncover important information that people do not know about their doctors, drug companies, and up-coming controversial technologies in order to hold Big Pharma accountable. The controversy and corruption that surrounds drug companies is immense.

Due to rising concerns and discussions about designer drugs, there is a failure of communication and unification among researchers concerning the profitability of them. Clinical trials are completed to ensure that drugs are safe and to ensure that they have the intended effects on patients. However, there are companies that skip this time and money consuming process in order to distribute their drugs sooner and make more money. Patents are put on drugs to protect drug companies from others producing and distributing their products. Drug Companies are now finding ways of making spiritual or magical treatments patentable and later trying to reach an incorrect conclusion as to why the treatment works in order to make more money. Again, concerns of money are high on the list of the drug companies. Pharmaceutical companies fail to focus on the patients and consequently put them in harm's way. Big Pharma's failure to unify and their running of corrupt clinical trials contribute to harming patients.

DRUG DESIGN AND DESIGNER DRUGS

Over the past five years, debates about designer drugs have been growing. This new sector's main focus is to genetically alter drugs so that they are custom for the individual patient. Although in theory this sounds like a health-improving technology, the failure of the multiple companies to agree on a destination and move forward is slowing the process, and as a result, is withholding treatment from patients that may save their lives. The rising issue of this new technology among the industry is the economic and marketing aspects of the drugs. The failure to unify and communicate among various sectors of this new field is harming the patients.

The business and marketing aspects are also in debate along with how the drugs should be designed. Hedgecoe and Martin, professors at Cardiff University, state that "the validity and clinical utility of the technology will have to be demonstrated, and commercially attractive products and services will need to be developed" (2013, p. 333). If a drug is safe and effective, it will sell itself. Drug companies spend 24.4% of their incoming money on promotions and only 13.4% on research ("Big Pharma Spends", 2008). TV commercials and free samples do not get the consumer to obtain the drug. The doctor writes a prescription if the doctor feels it is necessary and appropriate for the patient to be taking the drug, he/she will prescribe it. The commercial has no purpose and the sample simply is given from the doctor to the patient so they can try the medication and see if they react to it. The marketing of drugs is a waste of time and money that could be put to use for researching and improving the health of patients.

CLINICAL TRIALS GONE WRONG

The sneaky relationship between researchers and drug companies taint the trials and therefore put the patient in danger. Borison and Diamond, two psychiatrists from the Medical College of Georgia, are in jail because of endangering the safety of multiple patients by tainting trials of over twenty drugs in order to receive hundreds of thousands of dollars from Big Pharma. Reuben, of Baystate Medical Center, is in prison for holding fraudulent trials for Celebrex®, Neurontin®, and Lyrica®. A Tucson facility held fixed trials for three asthma drugs to obtain $10,000 a patient from Big Pharma. The article published on *AlterNet* also released that Massachusetts General Hospital supported Johnson & Johnsons drug Risperdal® before the drug company even tested it (Rosenberg, 2010). Doctors, respected pillars of the medical profession cheated the public out of their health for their own personal short-term benefits. Once again the power of money overpowers people's judgments in the pharmaceutical industry.

Gender Inequality

The purpose of conducting clinical trials is to make sure that the drugs are safe and do what the researchers expect. In the 1920s and 1930s, Organon, a Netherland pharmaceutical company, was involved in the development of hormonal drugs. The first drug that was produced and distributed was called Menformon, a female sex hormone. This sex hormone was tested among five people. Not only was it a small test group, the group consisted of Laqueur and four of his colleagues at the Pharmaco-Therapeutic Laboratory in Amsterdam. Shortly after the scientists tried the drug, it was marketed and sold. Organon and Laqueur debated if the clinical trials should be done before the drug was released, but decided it was not necessary to wait for the results because of the competition surrounding the new drug. In a letter that Laqueur wrote to Organon that was published in the Organon archive on December 12, 1925, Laqueur states:

We can only learn by experience whether female sex hormone therapy will be of any clinical value… Theoretically, one cannot make the slightest prediction whether it will have any useful effects. In the end this will have to appear in practice.

(qtd. in Oudshoorn, 1993, p. 11)

The only clinical trials that were done were from males using the drug and there were no controls implemented to eliminate biases. It was not a true clinical trial because nothing was documented except the results. Their "clinical trials" were not only limited, but extremely inaccurate and therefore impossible to draw scientific conclusions from.

The male sex hormone was not put onto the market until five years after the female sex hormone. One may argue that it is sexist releasing the female's hormone before the male's, and having more testing done for the male's treatment than the female's treatment. Organon released a statement that included the following: "It is not the task of the pharmaceutical industry to restrain the marketing of a much requested product" (Oudshoorn, 1993, p. 17). They are indeed responsible for the well-being of their consumers and need to be aware of the safety of the substance they are administering. It is not just a matter of courtesy; it is a moral and ethical issue. It is their job. The minds of the companies are focused so heavily on profit margins that they fail to acknowledge the life behind the number.

The Rights of Patients

The lack of requirements of clinical trials is killing patients. A mother in Minnesota lost her son to suicide due to his involuntary participation in a psychiatric drug study at the University of Minnesota. The university was receiving a profit from a pharmaceutical company to hold the trial. The drug led her son to suicide. It all started with him changing his last name, and then placing objects around his bed to protect him from devils, and later threats of slicing his mother's throat and delusions of being convinced that the Illuminati were creating a storm in Duluth where he would kill people that he was told to murder. It ended with him stabbing "himself to death in the bathtub with a box cutter, ripping open his abdomen and nearly decapitating himself," the mother "literally fell to her knees and started to shriek and cry" when she received the news (Elliott, 2010). The selfishness of these drug companies is taking lives.

Overseas in Nigeria, children died while participating in trials involving Trovan®, an antibiotic used to treat respiratory, stomach, and urinary tract infections. Pfizer, the maker of Trovan®, paid the government of Nigeria millions of dollars as part of a settlement. Pfizer also tried to drop the charges by extorting Nigeria's former attorney general (Rosenberg, 2010). Pharmaceutical companies look for poor countries to help test their products. In doing so, sometimes the drug company kills thousands of people. Drug companies do not care about the patient's life, they just want their money at whatever cost and are willing to lose a little of it to gain much more.

The pure corruption that surrounds the field is astounding. The National Association for Rights Protection and Advocacy (NARPA) reports that twenty percent of children who have visited a psychiatrist left with a prescription for a drug even though many reports of side-effects were released (Elliott, 2010). Companies also cover up data and make the unfavorable results look less significant than they are. Some studies are even hidden from the FDA so a drug receives approval. By companies funding commercials, releasing drugs early, and gaining the approval of doctors, Big Pharma gets the FDA to approve drugs that should not be approved. Trials that are financed by drug companies skew the results to make their drugs look favorable. Faking positives and skewing data is not what medicine is. The drug industry has become a mean and aggressive institution that has embraced competition with every brain cell of their body to profit in any way they possibly can.

Maintaining the Order

The whole purpose of clinical trials is to ensure comprehensive testing of new drugs before they become available to the general public. Due to the design of the trial phases, the intent is that the phases should be executed sequentially. This means that each phase is meant to find more and more issues with the drug (Herper, 2016a). If a drug can't pass Phase I, it won't be able to pass Phase II.

An experimental anti-depressant made by Alkermes is being discussed at the FDA. In Phase II, the study was successful; however the drug was only tested in a small group of people and the results were not statistically significant. Alkermes' CEO, Richard Pops, argues that "earlier studies" were consistent with this Phase II. Guidance from the FDA agrees with Pops, "because of the big placebo effects in depression studies, even effective drugs will fail half the time. But the requirement for approval has always been two successful late-stage, or Phase III studies, no matter how many fail" (Herper, 2016a). This line of thinking was also apparent in a Parkinson's drug, Nuplazid (Acadia Pharmaceuticals), where it failed in one trial, passed in a second trial, and the FDA approved the drug.

Another example is the approval of a drug even though it only resulted in raising a protein level minimally. That company's hope was that it could use the approved drug to test the broader affected population. This unethical behavior has gotten to the point where companies are trying to use one successful Phase III trial to justify a piece of previous studies. This justification of the FDA approval process is convoluted and harmful to the patients that may ultimately take a given drug: A drug doesn't really pass in Phase II, but it's pushed to Phase III to prove Phase II was a success. Breaking the sequential order of clinical trials is risky behavior in the regulatory process and needs to be stopped.

SUGAR PILLS

Placebos are commonly viewed as fraud among the general public. Some news stories have said that some drugs that were sold as prescriptions were just milk and sugar. Although it is wrong to sell placebos in place of real drugs, placebos have a great deal of importance in pharmaceutical research. Placebos can make a control group stronger. Using placebos allow the control group to not get the actual drug to prevent the consumer from knowing if he/she actually received a drug or not. This can lessen surrounding biases. However, recent discoveries are showing that some placebos are working better than real drugs.

An article in *Wired* reports that from 2001 to 2006 the percentage of products that failed Phase II clinical trials rose by twenty percent (Silberman, 2009). Half of all drugs that fail in late-stage trials drop out of the pipeline due to their inability to beat sugar pills. The drug developers claim that the placebo effect is somehow getting stronger. The placebo has and will be the same for years to come just as it has stayed the same all through the years before. Milk and sugar, is milk and sugar. The decrease in new drugs is due to the failure to meet the FDA standard that a new medication must beat a placebo in at least two trials. This further demonstrates that Big Pharma is so busy thinking of ways to earn money that they have lost their ability to make new innovative drugs and improve the industry. The distractions of money affect Big Pharma's ability to do their job: helping people.

Alternative Medicine

Since drugs are becoming less effective and companies are running out of new drugs, practitioners are exploring the field of alternative medicine. They are not only researching it, they are twisting it so that they can find connections to science to make it patentable and profitable. The field of alternative medicine in Tibet is becoming more of an interest to many in the drug industry. It has become a race to get the patent, but in order to do that, researchers must "[push] that which is deemed spiritual or magical either out of the picture or into a form that is biological" (Adams, 2002, p. 679). Big Pharma companies are so desperate and are running out of ideas that they have to merge other fields and reach for conclusions that look scientific.

MONETARY SETTLEMENTS

With all of the settlements that Big Pharma has to pay, one might conclude that the industry is not stable enough to support itself; however, drug companies are experiencing growth and are commonly found on the Fortune 500 List (Law, 2006). According AlterNet, "Pharmaceutical companies have been hit with $14.8 billion in wrongdoing settlements in the last five years. But that's still cheaper for Big Pharma than going about things the old-fashioned, legal way. So the fraud continues" (Rosenberg, np, 2010). Compared to what drug companies make annually, their settlements are a mere fine. An AstraZeneca settlement was $302 million because they were paying doctors to prescribe

Seroquel®, an anti-psychotic drug, for unapproved uses. The one-time fee of $302 million dollars does not compare to their annual income of $32.8 billion. A Pfizer settlement was $2.3 billion for violations of the Food, Drug and Cosmetic Act due to excessively prescribing Bextra®, a painkiller, for uses not approved by the FDA. The $2.3 billion settlement is a rarity, but Pfizer is a larger company that makes $50 billion annually (Landman, 2010).

One of the smaller settlements was a Johnson & Johnson settlement for $700,000, which was the most severe in terms of health endangerment but yet the lowest in numerical value. Information about Levaquin® was withheld from the public; Levaquin® is a bacterial infection antibiotic. The settlement included over 2,600 claims surrounding Levaquin® (Llamas, 2016). On top of the settlement being one of the smallest and encompassing the numerous claims, Johnson & Johnson makes around $61.89 billion.

Pharmaceutical Companies fail to acknowledge the well-being of their patients and in-turn fail to treat them to the capabilities that modern technology allows. Hedgecoe and Martin (2013) examine the two visions that are emerging within the pharmaceutical industry. A field of study that researches and implements trials around genetically personalized drugs is forming in the mist of debate and controversy. Their essay explores the field of pharmacogenetics and how it has two possible ways of developing into an industry that can reduce the number of adverse drug reactions (ADRs). The way in which scientists are striving to achieve this is in one of two ways: either 1. study the genetic make-up of diseases and alter the drugs accordingly, or 2. study the patient's genome and make a drug solely for them. The goal of distributing personalized drugs to patients is to reduce the side-effects which will lower the number of low suits against drug companies.

Dirty Suits

Moderna is a drug company that's been very secretive about what product they're developing. The startup claims to be working on a new class of drugs that manipulate antibodies into producing drugs via therapeutic proteins (Vardi, 2016). It wasn't until Acuitas filed a lawsuit in British Columbia that Moderna revealed exactly what they're working on. Acuitas licensed a technology to Moderna that they don't own. A third company, Arbutus, owns the technology and decided to terminate the license. Acuitas thought that by filing a lawsuit, they could protect the deal they had with Moderna. This triggered Arbutus to countersue and claim its deal with Acuitas didn't cover the deal between Moderna and Acuitas. In the end, Moderna settled on three different drug technology methods, one for each company. Then Moderna turned back to Acuitas to gain access to the technology that Arbutus owned. Licensing, sublicensing, lawsuits, and countersuits demonstrate the length that Big Pharma will go to undercut each other and generate revenue for themselves.

A new initiative of the FDA to get more drugs reviewed is the granting of a Priority Review Voucher (PRV). If a drug company gets approval for one of their drugs that treat certain rare pediatric diseases, they are granted a transferrable voucher to expedite the FDA's review of a future drug (Jarvis, 2015a). In 2015, two PRVs were used to speed up the approval of highly anticipated drugs. Sanofi used a PRV to get their PCSK9 inhibitor approved a month ahead of Amgen's competing drug. On the surface, PRVs seem beneficial to getting drugs approved faster, but in reality they're fueling the crooked, under-handed moves of the industry.

Monetary Manipulation

On the surface, it may sometimes look like drug companies are doing good things with their money and trying to improve the society that consumes their products. Nestle, a candy company based in Switzerland, is partnering with a drug company to provide its food engineering expertise in a joint effort to make medicines taste good. For years, candy companies disbursed their unhealthy, sugary products through society subsequently making people diabetic, obese, and depressed. With the increase in nutrition education, sugar restrictions imposed by governments, and people being generally more health-conscious, candy companies like Nestle are experiencing an all-time low period of sales. This is what has caused Nestle to enter the drug flavoring sector. "If making consumers fat has been big business, making them healthy could be bigger" (Campbell & Gretler, 2016). Big Pharma's intention is always related to making money.

LIMITING ACCESS TO INCREASE PROFIT

Views on antibiotics have changed over the years. It used to be that the standard was to have doctors prescribe antibiotics for the littlest ailments. Now, doctors are to be more cautious when prescribing antibiotics and only prescribe them if it's absolutely necessary. For antibiotics, it's beneficial for pharmaceutical companies to limit the drug's effectiveness so that the bacteria is eliminated at a level that doesn't produce symptoms in the patient, but isn't eliminated from the patient completely. This causes patients to get "cured" and then treated again and that cycle continues (Altstedter & Trivedi, 2017). At the same time, it can spread to other patients. Big Pharma has no incentive to cure people. The profits are in treatment options because patients have to consistently receive medication.

The reasoning for the need to decrease the distribution of antibiotics is because bacteria can become resistant overtime if they have more opportunities to encounter the drugs. This has happened in India and is becoming a major public health issue. Medical experts believe the nation has one of the highest levels of drug-resistant tuberculosis in the world (Altstedter & Trivedo, 2017). As a result, Prime Minister Modi enacted regulation to preserve the effectiveness of bedaquiline, a drug used to treat tuberculosis.

In India, the drug can only be dispensed through a government program as a last treatment option.

On one side, the effectiveness of drugs needs to be maintained not only for being able to treat the sickest patients, but also to prolong the period of time that Big Pharma can profit from their latest drug discoveries. Ramanan Laxminarayan, a senior research scholar at Princeton, says that "It's a public health issue that we get to control access to this drug, make sure someone who is absolutely dying of extensively drug-resistant tuberculosis is the one who gets to have it" (Altstedter & Trivedo, 2017). On the other hand, patients need to have access to certain life-saving drugs. Jennifer Furin, a lecturer at Harvard Medical School, believes that India is turning medical issues into bureaucratic issues (Altstedter & Trivedo, 2017).

NARCOTIC FENTANYL AND BRIBING

The prescribing of fentanyl is highly regulated by the FDA as it's a scheduled II drug. This means that it's rather addictive and subject to abuse. Some pharmaceutical companies are seeking to enter this market by formulating the drug in different forms of administration (ie: spray, injection, oral, etc.). Michael Babich from Insys Therapeutics was arrested for bribing doctors to prescribe Insys Therapeutics' mouth spray formulation of fentanyl (Herper, 2016b). The oral spray is given under the patient's tongue and is absorbed quickly into the bloodstream to reduce pain. This is especially critical in patients that suffer from severe cancer pain.

Lastly, the indictment against Babich also proves evidence of giving prescribers monetary compensation in order to write prescriptions for Subsys®. During August 2012 to May 2015, Insys allegedly paid $731,475.07 to get doctors to speak on their behalf, and doctors wrote 7,974 prescriptions for Subsys®.

CONCLUSION

The combination of lousy settlements, the FDA passing suboptimal drugs, and the scarceness of new drugs allows Big Pharma to continue to carry out their agenda while not having to consider the needs of the patient. The entire healthcare system in general is broken. This is mostly due to failed policies; segmented markets and services; and a lack of consensus on how the system is to operate while pleasing the most stakeholders. The prescription industry has become corrupted due to the greedy agendas of Big Pharma executives. In theory, this smaller segment of the healthcare system should be easier to fix.

9

GlaxoSmithKline's Agenda

Companies looking to gain space in markets oversees need to be aware of local laws and regulations that are applicable to their industry. Companies that operate in China are subject to local laws and need to pay close attention to anti-bribery laws. GlaxoSmithKline is a multinational drug company that employs 100,000 people around the world (7,000 of which are located in China) and has achieved global sales over $22 billion (Quelch & Rodriguez, 2013). A scandal that GSK was involved in resulted in a settlement of $3 billion; it was the largest fraud scandal in the healthcare industry in US history. Bribery and scandals of foreign companies operating in China is not a rarity ("China Focus", 2012). GlaxoSmithKline's ethics policy was good at providing a framework for the organization to abide by; however, there is much work that GSK can do in order to prevent the China bribery scandal from happening again.

GSK'S ETHICS AND COMPLIANCE PROGRAM

Organizations of all shapes and sizes usually have a compliance program, especially if they directly report to or are reimbursed by a federal institution. Typically a code of ethics is a part of that program. A study from the Society of Corporate Compliance and Ethics (SCCE) found that only 47% of companies distribute their code of ethics and only 26% require certification that the policy has been read (Jaeger, 2009). A policy does not serve its full potential if it is left unread. It's recommended that companies share these policies with third-parties that interact with the business.

One of the initiatives GSK had in place was an ethics policy that clearly states that its employees are to comply with the local laws in the regions in which they operate. Another initiative the drug company has taken is creating a "Speak Up Integrity" hotline. Numerous other companies have this as a medium for their employees to report instances of fraud, waste, and abuse in a confidential, safe, and anonymous environment. GSK also claims to have trained their employees in these topics. Even though a policy such as a Code of Ethics is implemented, it may be extremely hard to enforce and monitor (Lord, 2013). This is why oversight and enforcement bodies are crucial to the successful implementation of any policy.

WHAT WENT WRONG?

A lack of oversight could have led to the breaking of GSK's ethics policy. Even though a policy is in place, there needs to be careful monitoring and enforcement to maintain compliance. This is especially difficult when there are no transnational enforcement bodies (Lord, 2013). Perhaps hiring a daughter of a former Communist Party leader as the director of corporate affairs was a poor idea. A local resident should know the local laws; however, she probably is not familiar with the laws and customs of the US which GSK also has to abide by. As part of the scandal, GSK employees were accused of bribing physicians, hospital administrators, and government officials (Quelch & Rodriguez, 2013). Several factors contributed to the events that caused the GSK scandal in China.

External and Internal Factors to Facilitate Bribery

One factor that contributed to the GSK scandal in China is that the top Big Pharma companies dominate large amounts of shares in China's market. This leads to great competition. The locally based drug companies do not have to follow US laws like GSK does. Also, for local drug companies in China, it is commonplace to bribe hospital staff. Some local universities go as far as classifying these actions as a "common marketing strategy" (Quelch & Rodriguez, 2013). China has provisions against bribery but it is commonplace in business transactions. Lastly, the fact that China is a monopolized sector with a lack of transparency also aided the bribery to occur ("China Focus", 2012). An increase in transparency led by enforcement bodies could have helped in the prevention of the GSK scandal in China.

In general, the adjustment to cultural differences can be difficult. Daniels, Radebaugh, & Sullivan state that there are four issues when adjusting to cultural differences:

- Extent to which a culture is willing to accept the introduction of anything foreign
- Whether key cultural differences are small or great
- The ability of individuals to adjust to what they find in foreign cultures
- The general management orientation of the company involved

(2015)

The issue that really applies to the GSK scandal is the ability of individuals to adjust to what they find in foreign cultures. It seems as though the GSK employees have adjusted too well. GSK adjusted so well that they became involved in local, illegal bribery activities. Some other political and legal factors for international business operations surround constructs of culture, economy, and geography, but most importantly, political and legal factors which plagued GSK. The role of government in society, political ideologies, political risk, the legal environment, and strategic legal issues all contributed to the events that led up to the GSK scandal (Daniels et al., 2015). Given all of these factors to monitor, it is extremely important to have a strong, knowledgeable team in place to combat negative events such as this one.

ASSESSMENT OF GSK'S RESPONSE AND PREVENTATIVE MEASURES

The ethics policy is a start, but there are still numerous things that GSK could have done to prevent this from happening. Having training in ethics and Chinese customs could have helped GSK in the prevention of this scandal. Also, improvement to the existing measures should be done. The fraud, waste, and abuse hotline that GSK setup could allow for more transparency between workers and managers. In terms of settlement, GSK paid out money under terms of an agreement with the US FDA for marketing drugs for unapproved indications and bribing doctors (Quelch & Rodriguez, 2013). This is not only extremely unethical, but also illegal. If GSK would have held themselves to a higher standard, the entire scandal could have been avoided.

GSK's General Manager in China

The general manager for GSK in China, Mark Reilly, should have been involved more in his organization and had crisis contingency policies in place. Modes of communication, template responses, and chains of command should have been established way before this ever happened. His role is even more important now in order to lead GSK and prevent this situation from ever happening again. Mark Reilly's role in China is vital to the prevention of future scandals like this. The scandal could be an opportunity for GSK to improve the organizational structure of the company so that it can handle this situation better in the future.

GSK's Defense

GSK was treated unfairly. Marketing drugs for unapproved indications has enormous implications on patient safety and raises grave legal concerns. Even though GSK engaged in irreprehensible conduct, they were simply acting as they saw others do in the corporate world in China. In the end, GSK should have familiarized themselves with Chinese custom and business laws. Perhaps doing so would have prevented this unfortunate situation. On the other hand, with lots of competition in the market and seeing how the locals conduct business, it is understandable how GSK got caught up in the scandal. Although it is understandable how GSK's organization contained loopholes to allow the bribery to occur, that does not mean that they cannot or should not be held responsible for their poor judgment.

STRATEGY AND OPERATIONS

GSK has an internal audit program in place. It confirmed that the 4 employees detained by the Chinese government had in fact engaged in fraud and bribery (Quelch & Rodriguez, 2013). They should have reacted sooner, by doing so, they could have avoided the entire scandal and all of the negative publicity that ensued as a result. A great example of prevention, strategy, and operations when a company is in the midst of a scandal is the company Siemens. The new CEO of Siemens, Peter Löscher, joined the company when they were under major scrutiny by numerous governmental bodies. Peter Löscher took on the position with great initiative. He noticed that employees didn't know each other's roles and responsibilities (Löscher, 2012). He immediately reorganized the entire organization so that upper management and lower management would be integrated better. He increased diversity, brought a new perspective (he was the only external hire as CEO since the founding of the company in 1847), and revamped the company's mission to be more customer-driven. By reducing bureaucracy, reorganizing the company, and centering its values, Peter Löscher led Siemens out of a bribery crisis similar to that of GSK.

U. S. FOREIGN CORRUPT PRACTICES ACT AND THE U.K. BRIBERY ACT

There are two major pieces of legislation in the US and abroad that are relevant to the GSK scandal: the Foreign Corrupt Practices Act (FCPA) and the UK Bribery Act. The FCPA defines bribery as illegal payments to foreign officials, political parties, party officials, and political candidates (Daniels et al., 2015). The UK Bribery Act is a bit more specific. It offers guidance on how UK companies can implement procedures that combat bribery. There is also an organization in the UK that works with the Attorney General and prosecutes those who commit bribery and corruption. This has proven useful in catching illegal business transactions at home and abroad.

Bold statements made by GSK's management displayed the efforts of mending the company's international relations with the locals. Hussain, the international president of Europe, Japan, emerging markets, and Asia Pacific, of GSK, "promised that GSK would partner with the Chinese government to remedy the situation" (Quelch & Rodriguez, 2015, p. 7). He also promised to make drugs less costly for Chinese consumers. Mark Reilly was replaced by Herve Gisserot as the GSK general manager of China. China does not have specific laws to combat bribery like the United States' FCPA or the UK's Bribery Act ("China Focus", 2012). China subscribes to a mixture of civil law and customary law (Daniels et al., 2015). Civil Law relies on tradition and established case law. Customary Law relies on the strength of a community and recognizing the benefits of compliance with established community standards. Politics inside and outside of GSK played roles in the developments of the GSK bribery scandal.

RECOMMENDATIONS

There is a severe lack of laws, oversight, monitoring, and enforcement in instances surrounding fraud, waste, and abuse. There are great improvements to be had. First there can be an international enforcement body that sets standards for conducting international business. The enforcement body would set new laws, require businesses to engage in training, and monitor transactions to detect fraud, waste, and abuse. Another problem lies in communication within a company across its multiple locations. Pfizer had an allegation against them and claimed that its management in the US was unaware of the actions and approvals that led up to their scandal ("China Focus", 2012). Companies need to ensure that they are talking internally across geographical locations. Most of the time, there are teams that are spread between offices. There needs to be a team that handles communications and has one representative from each plant to distribute updates company-wide.

LESSONS LEARNED

Out of misfortune comes a learning opportunity. Lessons learned can be useful for GSK going forward. Shobert and DeNoble recommend that the industry needs to be redefined and laws need to be stricter. Some suggested improvements are:

1. Revenue growth expectations for the Chinese market need to be tempered
2. The room for discretionary spending – especially non-receipted travel and entertainment expenses – has grown markedly narrower
3. When problems present themselves – and they most certainly will as new standards and expectations are rolled out – make a point of communicating the punishment to your China sales force

4.   Re-configure how your sales force sells
5.   Increase compliance staffing levels
6.   Payments to third parties such as industry organizations, affiliate networks, and event organizers need to be audited
7.   Make sure distributors understand your compliance standards and that they are following your lead in terms of how their sales force is trained, audited, and incentivized
8.   Make an effort to apologize

(2013)

Those lessons learned are based in logic and legal consequences. There must be a shift in focus regarding internal control of an organization's ethics; changing from an ideology of how to legally comply, to one that is concerned with how to satisfy Chinese authorities. Organizations that are action-oriented instead of legally-oriented will achieve success. GSK's issue seems to lie in the enforcement and monitoring of those written documents.

CONCLUSION

GSK had a policy in place to prevent the China bribery scandal from occurring, but there is obviously room for improvement. GSK is not the only drug company to be involved in a scandal like this. AstraZeneca, UCB, Novo Nordisk, and Lundbeck have also been investigated by the Chinese government (Quelch & Rodriguez, 2013).

Allegations of bribery and marketing unapproved drug indications have surfaced as a result of these investigations. Patterns of these investigations suggest that it is common for the drug company to just pay settlements rather than admit to wrongdoings. A shift in thinking is occurring in the Chinese government regarding bribery and who is responsible. They used to prosecute the person accepting the bribe, now they are looking more at the person offering the bribe. There is great improvement that is needed in order to prevent this type of corporate misconduct in the future.

10

Big Cost

Big Pharma is a dynamic and complex industry. Just a few of the stakeholders include researchers, drug companies, pharmacies, governmental agencies, health plans, doctors, and patients. Agencies such as the Food and Drug Administration (FDA), National Institutes of Health (NIH), Department of Health, and the Drug Enforcement Agency (DEA) have much influence on the pharmaceutical industry in America. One doesn't have to look far to start to understand how the health and drug industry became so convoluted. All of the stakeholders in the industry have a role in cleaning up the system and ensuring patients get the drugs that they desperately need. Looking back at the drug approvals during the past three years, the types of drugs vary greatly. In 2014, forty-one drugs were approved (8 cancer drugs, 17 orphan drugs), the majority being antibodies, peptides, and enzymes (Jarvis, 2015b). In 2015, thirty-eight drugs were approved

(13 cancer drugs, 12 antibodies and peptides), the majority being small molecules. Harvoni® (Gilead Sciences) took the spotlight with $13.9 billion in sales, a 554% increase from 2014 (Thayer, 2015).

The big pharmaceutical industry comes with a big price tag. Big Pharma doesn't seem to care about the millions of patients behind the billions of dollars. Research, development, and marketing costs are indeed expensive, but not nearly as expensive as the cost of the drugs they sell. The top nine most expensive drugs, on average, cost more than $200,000 a year for each patient that takes them (Herper, 2010). The majority of these drugs treat rare, genetic diseases that affect fewer than 10,000 patients. This is the main reason Big Pharma can basically charge whatever they want. The fewer the patients affected, the higher the demand, the more Big Pharma can charge.

TRENDS IN DRUG PRICING

The world's most expensive drug, as of 2016, is Soliris® (Alexion Pharmaceuticals) being priced at $409,500 a year per patient. The disease that this drug treats only affects 8,000 Americans, but the drug maker generated $295 million in one year for that one drug (Herper, 2010). Drug pricing is largely based on the number of people who have the disorder: as the number of people affected by the disorder increases, the drug price decreases. Initially Soliris® was tested for treating patients with Rheumatoid

Arthritis (RA). If it would've been FDA approved for treating RA, it would've cost $20,000 a year per patient. Since the drug was approved for treating Paroxysmal Nocturnal Hemoglobinuria (PNH), which only affects 8,000 Americans, it's priced at $409,500 per patient per year.

The prices of these new drugs that treat rare diseases seem to increase every year. A long time ago they were $100,000 per year per patient. Now, that is typical of any drug's price (Herper, 2010). Since there are only a few patients in need of these drugs, Big Pharma doesn't need to advertise these drugs because the government and insurance companies typically pay for the drugs. However, there is hope on the horizon. Since Pfizer and other companies are awaiting FDA approval for similar drugs that treat these rare diseases, competition will enter the market soon and drive down these astronomical prices.

PRICING INJUSTICES

Epi-Pen
A very recent point of contention is the price of Epi-Pens® (Mylan). Epi-Pens® save the lives of people who experience anaphylactic shocks. Due to numerous petitions, Mylan claims that they dropped the price of the Epi-Pen®. But in reality, Mylan simply offered a $300 savings card to underinsured consumers ("The Other 98%", 2017). Everyone else, even if they're on Medicare or Medicaid, pays the full price of $600. Mylan only offered a temporary

Band-Aid solution to the price controversy. If the FDA were to breakup Mylan's monopoly of the Epi-Pen®, it would make quality healthcare a right, rather than a privilege. Auvi-Q® (Kaléo), an alternative to the Epi-Pen®, contains auto-injector technology and actually instructs the user how to administer the medication. This is a great way to help patients safely administer the life-saving medication; however, this greatly impacts the price of the drug. The company's CEO claims that they're still "working with stakeholders to set the price" (Bonner, 2017). The company claims to remain committed to lowering the most important price: the price to the patient.

If patient's still are not able to afford the Epi-Pen® or Auvi-Q®, there is a generic alternative: epinephrine auto-injector. It is important that patients and prescribers are aware that the FDA does not consider the generic alternative to be equivalent to the Epi-Pen® or Auvi-Q®. This forces doctors to have to explicitly write on the prescription "epinephrine auto-injector". This requirement is commonly overlooked as "Epi-Pen®" has become the generally accepted term for any kind of epinephrine pen.

The Convoluted Insulin Monopoly

Looking back in time, it's mind-boggling to think about how Big Pharma pricing became so far out of control. Insulin therapy, presently in mainstream high supply and demand, used to be a cutting-edge treatment that was difficult to create. The three person team that created a way to generate insulin recognized the need for this thera-py and wanted to ensure the public could access it safely. They put their words into motion and sold the patent for in-sulin to the University of Toronto for $1 ("Insulin's Inventor Sold the Patent", 2017). The university, years later, gave the rights royalty-free to Big Pharma. At the time, Banting and his team just wanted it available for the public good and thought that by not charging royalties to Big Pharma, they'd keep the prices low. In the meantime, the process-ing of synthetic insulin was perfected making it easier to produce, and the price increased. Green and Riggs state:

> The history of insulin highlights the limits of generic competition as a public-health framework. Nearly a century after its discovery, there is still no inexpensive supply of insulin for people living with diabetes in North America, and Americans are paying a steep price for the continued rejuvenation of the oldest of modern medicines.
> ("Insulin's Inventor Sold the Patent", np, 2017)

This further demonstrates that no one should ever under-estimate the power of Big Pharma.

Other Costly Drugs
The news and media have paid attention to and have heav-ily scrutinized the price inflation of the Epi-Pen®. Parallel to that media aversion, is the price inflation of Daraprim®.

Daraprim® is used to treat a parasitic infection. The drug maker raised the price from $15 to $750 resulting in a 5,000% increase in price. Valeant Pharmaceuticals did something similar with Isuprel® and Nitropress®, medications for the heart; they raised the price 500% and 200% respectively (Mullin, 2015). The question society seems to be asking is shifting from "wow isn't that drug amazing?" to "How can I afford it?". A positive shift in drug pricing is on the horizon.

THE MEDIATOR ROLE OF THE PBM

Some critics of industry prices think the high prices are due to pharmacy benefit managers (PBM). PBMs are essentially the middleman between the pharmacy and the drug manufacturer. However, as Tim Wentworth, a CEO from Express Scripts states, "Drug makers set prices, and we [the PBM] exist to bring them down" (Weinberg & Langreth, 2017). About 60 years ago, PBMs started as just payment processers. Now PBMs create formularies and negotiate prices with pharmacies, insurance companies, and manufacturers. Even though in some instances PBMs pocket manufacturer rebates, charge insurance companies more for generics, and funnel patients to their own specialty and mail-order pharmacies, PBMs have successfully decreased medication costs in areas such as Hepatitis C. PBMs sit opportunistically between drug manufactures and insurance plans which allows them to increase competition between equivalent drugs and drive prices down.

Regulation's Role

Some argue that it was too much regulation, not too little regulation that has caused the FDA to reject competing drugs due to existing patents. In a sense, this is good so that pharmaceutical companies can recoup R&D costs to create new drugs. On the other hand, the patients need to be able to afford the existing drugs (Fox, 2016). The industry tries to remediate this catch 22 by issuing patents. These temporary monopolies allow Big Pharma to set the price; then upon patent expiration, competition ensues. Because of this current model, a new type of drug company is emerging: a drug company doesn't create drugs, but rather takes advantage of existing drugs with expired patents. Perhaps a solution to the drug pricing problem is to increase competition.

THE FIX

If the system isn't entertaining a solution to decrease drug costs, a solution can be implemented to decrease medical costs. Dr. Barbara McAneny, CEO of the New Mexico Cancer Center, has demonstrated that it's possible to decrease costs while improving patient care. Appropriately prioritizing care via comprehensive triage and treatment decision trees can decrease the number of costly Emergency Room (ER) visits. Also, aggressively managing side-effects of cancer drug therapies can aid in this decrease of ER visits. The more that cancer patients can avoid the ER, the better, as immune compromised cancer patients should not be around sit patients (McAneny, 2016). Extended clinician office hours can aid in patients seeking medication or emergency care. Prioritization, pathways, and extended office hours can get patients treated more effectively and timely which ultimately reduces costs.

Doctor and patients don't have the power to influence market share. A few broad solutions to decrease cost and improve patient care include:

- Holding retail chains responsible for patient adherence
- Implementing value-based contracting with pharmacies
- Specialized pharmacy care to increase adherence and improves health outcomes
- Adding utilization management programs on formularies to decrease the cost to patients and insurers

(Miller, 2017)

There is a growing gap between a drug's list price and the net price. This has been caused by closed formularies which increase member's out-of-pocket costs (Gottlieb, 2017). The federal government is increasingly becoming a payer for prescription drugs. Washington can address the issues around drug pricing by increasing product and price competition.

Biosimilar Drugs

Biosimilar drugs are identical copies of a product that has an expired patent. They are expected to increase competition and reduce drug prices. Europe, Canada, Japan, and Australia have sold dozens of biosimilar drugs for ten years. In the US, prices are expected to drop by 35%. In addition, $80 billion in sales will lose patent protection through 2020 (Thayer, 2015). In 2015, $10 billion in sales already lost their patent protection. In 2016, sales for biologics drastically beat out the sales of small molecules. The drug with the most sales was Humira with $16.1 billion in sales, a 13% increase from 2015 (Thayer, 2017). New biosimilar drugs and other specialty drugs are increasingly coming to market; however, they still look economically like brand drugs. The Pharmacy Benefit Manager (PBM) sits opportunistically to profit from rebates and formulary placement (Hill, 2017). Oddly enough, the Federal Government does not determine which drugs are biosimilar, the PBM does. The industry needs to be mindful of where prescriptions are coming from (ie: specialty doctor, primary care provider, etc.) as that also dictates the price.

Value-based Contracting

Value-based contracting helps hold Big Pharma accountable. If the drug shows a lack of clinical effectiveness and/or results in unreported side effects, the manufacture owes the plan sponsor two-thirds of the drug's cost. Rishi Manchanda, the Chief Medical Officer (CMO) of

The Wonderful Company, believes that the sequel to the triple aim is the quadruple aim which is comprised of: outcomes, costs, provider experience, and patient experience (Manchanda, 2016). The downside of this approach is that if a drug doesn't work, the insurance company gets a "penalty fee" from the drug manufacturer. So essentially what is happening is that if ineffective drugs are administered to patients, meaning that the patient is not getting better or is even getting worse, the insurance company profits (Appleby, 2017). One on hand the insurance company may need the extra money to subsequently care for the patient, but it seems like the insurance company will always profit in the end. The rising cost of prescription drugs is unsustainable. Value-based contracts can add both financial and therapeutic value.

Formulary Administration

Some other ways to manage cost include: intelligent purchasing, real-time surveillance, and versatile cost management strategies (Allemand, 2017). Comprehensive formularies, pharmacy networks, and clinical care are also ways to lower healthcare costs. A common mistake made by health insurance companies is that they setup their formularies based on the drug. However, this leads to an increase in cost due to a lack of biosimilar drugs. When insurance companies segment their formularies based on indication, this decreases cost as there are more treatment options and more competition.

POWER OF THE PATIENT

From the perspective of the patient, there are a few ways they can try and save money on prescription drugs. For many expensive drugs, the manufacturer will have a savings card available. The card can usually be found on the manufacture's website or at the doctor's office. It's always a good idea to inquire at the pharmacy too. Some pharmacies have a savings program that can reduce the cost of generic medications. At the pharmacy counter, asking for a 90 day prescription can also reduce the out-of-pocket cost. When patients use in-network prescribers and in-network pharmacies, their costs can greatly decrease. Lastly, if a higher dosage of the same medication is cheaper than the prescribed dosage, the pharmacy can actually adjust the prescription so the patient can split the pills and save money (Kirchheimer, 2016).

If a patient is of the age to qualify for Medicare, there's a significant time of every year where the patient can take advantage of changing prescription insurance plans. This period is called Open Enrollment. Patients can re-evaluate their coverage and see if there are better plans that can save them money (Barry, 2016). Typically pharmacies will even run a report, upon request, to see which plan is the best based on the patient's medications. Usually this is a time where patients get frustrated that some of their medications or benefits are not covered anymore. This time can be taken advantage of to see if there are more cost-effective plans. When looking at insurance plans it's important to consider the following four C's: the cost of insurance, the convenience of in-network locations, the coverage of drugs and services, and the customer service that the plan provides ("Understanding Medicare", 2016). There are lots of solutions that patients have the power to take advantage of to save on the cost of medications.

CONCLUSION

The pharmaceutical market is simultaneously seeing an increase in cost of services and drug prices. This is the recipe for a perfect disaster. Big Pharma has lots of power when it comes to setting prices (Miller, 2017). The major diseases where drug price increases are seen include: diabetes, cancer, and multiple sclerosis (Allemand, 2017). This is also seen in Alzheimer's drugs. There still is not a proven treatment for Alzheimer's, but lots of people are affected by it. This gives Big Pharm the power to set the price. Another example is diabetes medications. The disease affects many patients, there is a severe lack of generics available, there are new treatments available, and insulin prices keep going up. Big Pharma takes advantage of the fact that it's hard to change insulin regimens and that doctors are reluctant to do so. Changing insulin regimes potentially involve an increase in drug usage, doctor visits, and overall costs. Don't be persuaded by Big Pharma's allure. Even if they rush a drug to market in an effort to supposedly improve access to needed medications, they most likely cut corners in their clinical trials and irresponsibly set the price of the drug.

11

The American Opioid Epidemic

The American Opioid Epidemic was a major topic of discussion of the twenty-first century. Opioid pain medication was being prescribed left-and-right. Initially, prescribers were being coached to prescribe more pain medication as pain was being greatly undertreated in patients. This was demonstrated in James Campbell's presidential address of the American Pain Society where he stated pain is the 5th vital sign (Waisbren, 2016). He urged the pharmacy profession to train doctors and nurses to treat pain by measuring it. Years later, there is a mixed consensus as to whether a physician tends to overprescribe opioids for chronic pain, or if physicians under-prescribe useful drugs for acute pain (Lichtblau, 1988). The Medical Board of Minnesota explicitly recommends that physicians adopt a multi-disciplinary approach to address all possible treatments to managing a patient's pain (Waisbren, 2016). Setting achievable, functional goals can help remediate therapeutic approaches to pain management. Even though the fault ultimately falls on the prescriber, it is important to note that prescribers take the advice of their medical societies and boards (Waisbren, 2016).

THE NUMBERS

The leading cause of death among 15-24 year olds is behavioral health problems (ie: substance abuse, mental health problems, risky sexual activity, etc.). Substance abuse seems to peak around people in their twenties and declines after that. According to "Facing Addiction in America", a report from the office of the Surgeon General, 20.8 million people over the age of 11 in 2015 had a substance use disorder (U.S. Department of Health and Human Services, 2016). That's 1.5 times the annual occurrence of all cancers combined. In 2015, more than 66 million people reported binge drinking and 27.1 million used illegal drugs. In 2014, around 45,000 people died from a drug overdose; this is greater than any previous year on record. Substance abuse costs the US more than $440 billion a year due to increased crime, healthcare, and lost productivity. Other estimates show that the misuse of opioids cost the US $78 billion a year in healthcare, criminal acts, and lost productivity (Williams & Wilkins, 2016). Twenty-eight billion of that $78 billion (36%) is attributed to healthcare costs alone. Clearly something needs to be done to stop the increase in these usage and death rates along with the increased costs.

THE NEED

It is clear that these illicit substances are damaging not only to the user of the substance, but also their loved ones, the healthcare system, and the government as a whole. Efforts to fix the epidemic have slowly started, but it needs to be fixed now. Effectuating change is a lengthy, complicated process, but when lives are at stake due to a system failure, immediate action is warranted. It's understood that the problem wasn't created overnight so it won't be fixed overnight, but something can be done to stop the epidemic from affecting more people. The most recent data has demonstrated that the problem is growing (U.S. Department of Health and Human Services, 2016). Widespread education on this issue needs to occur as substance misuse and addiction are preventable, solvable problems. The population impacted by this has quadrupled since 1999 and only 1 in 5 people affected actually get treatment (U.S. Department of Health and Human Services, 2016). Parents, families, educators, health professionals, policy makers, researchers, and the community need to all engage in fixing the opioid epidemic because everyone has a role in both the problem, and the solution. With immediate education, regulation, and treatment, the epidemic can be slowed, if not stopped.

THE IMPACT

A mom and dad are passed out with a four year old in the backseat of a car. A woman is lying in a grocery aisle as her toddler cries. These are just a few of the effects that the American Opioid Epidemic has had on children. According to hospital discharge papers, 13,052 children were hospitalized due to opioid poisonings between 1997 and 2012 (Cha, 2016). It seems significant to mention that overdoses in toddlers were accidental (ie: medicine cabinets not being child-proofed), whereas overdoses in kids more than 10 years old were attributed to attempts of suicide. On the surface, these numbers appear to have recently decreased. However, when researchers analyzed these trends separately, it was discovered that as prescription overdoses decreased, illicit drug overdoses increased (Cha, 2016). This aligns with the increase in difficulty in getting prescription drugs, and the increased use of illicit drugs in adults. For some patients, physical therapy is just not enough (Balick, 2016). In order to increase their quality of life, the pain itself needs to be treated (Cha, 2016).

ACTION TAKEN

In 2017, the FDA restricted the manufacturing of Schedule II Opiates by 25%. Obviously the FDA has a critical role in controlling the manufacturing quotas of Schedule I and II substances. When setting quotas, the institution did their due diligence in reviewing:

- Estimates of the legitimate medical need
- Estimates of retail consumption based on prescriptions dispensed
- Manufacturers' data on actual production, sales, inventory, exports, product development needs, and manufacturing losses
- Data from DEA's own internal system for tracking controlled substance transactions
- Past quota histories

(Balick, 2016)

Critics say that the FDA's reduced quota may lead to drug shortages for pain management and decrease access to other areas of pain management like oncology, hospice, and methadone clinics (Balick, 2016). Ab Osterhaus, a Dutch Professor, agrees that prescribers who write orders for inappropriate opioid treatments contribute to the problem (Balick, 2016). However, he believes that the DEA's guidelines are premature and won't be taken under advisement by practitioners immediately as there is not ample time for prescribers to transition patients to other pain management therapies.

FUTURE RECOMMENDATIONS

Substance abuse disorders were always undertreated. Although there has been an improvement in treatment due to increased education and research, there is still more that can be done. Only 10% of substance abuse patients receive specialized treatment (U.S. Department of Health and Human Services, 2016). Over 40% of patients with a substance abuse disorder also have a mental health condition. This treatment gap is due to the "inability to access or afford care, fear of shame and discrimination, and lack of screening for substance abuse disorders in healthcare settings" (U.S. Department of Health and Human Services, np, 2016). Multiple pain management methods are available as an alternative to controlling the opioid epidemic. Osterhaus advocates for a solution that doesn't put legitimate pain patients at risk, but rather focuses resources to prescribers and pharmacists. He encourages pharmacists to read the CDC's guidelines and be a resource to prescribers to improve patients' pain and quality of life (Balick, 2016).

12

Big, Idealistic Systems

Although there are lots of physical, tangible diseases that cause people to become ill, there is a single disease that is intangible, not quantifiable, but no less lethal. It's called Life Sucks Disease (LSD). People commonly accept the notion that high blood pressure, high cholesterol, and diabetes can kill us. But what about all of the other social factors that surround those diseases? Stressing about finances, work, and relationships can distract us all from the critical self-care that helps prevent things like high blood pressure, high cholesterol, and diabetes (Drane, 2016). Other symptoms of LSD include: cold sweats at kid's sports games, feeling that the weekend isn't long enough, and the temptation to call in sick (Schaefer, 2016). Physiologically, there is a reason that on Sundays, people fear the next day: Monday (Levitin, 2015). The amygdala gets activated and releases hormones in anticipation of the loss of freedom that comes with the start of the workweek. Other symptoms that can precipitate as a result of stress include: restlessness, sweating, muscle tension, and headaches.

Physicians need to ask probing questions to get patients to disclose these social stressors so that the whole patient can be treated. There are four things physicians can do: ask the patient probing questions, acknowledge the patient's hardships, connect with the patient, and treat the patient. Dr. Manchanda is already doing this. His upstream approach seeks to circumvent social and environmental issues before they lead to physical health problems (Manchanda, 2016). What happens outside the doctor's office is just as critical, if not more critical, than what goes on in the office. Issues in healthcare are typically indicative of systemic failures. Patients fall through the cracks for different reasons; however, odds are a single system failure does not just impact one patient. Health plans sit opportunistically between patients and care providers. They can use case management, care coordination, and analytics to ensure patients get optimal care that's delivered effectively.

THE "PARTS" OF MEDICARE

There are four "parts" to Medicare: Medicare Part A, Medicare Part B, Medicare Part C, and Medicare Part D. Part A covers stays in hospitals, long-term care facilities, hospice, and the medications that are administered in those care settings. Part B covers preventative screenings, test, counseling sessions, rehabilitation services, medical equipment, and vaccines and medications administered in the doctor's office. Medicare Part C is run by private insurance companies that determine benefit coverage for Parts A and Part B such as routine vision, hearing, and dental ("Understanding Medicare", 2016). Part C is comprised of private health plans (ie: HMOs and PPOs that cover Part D in one package). Part D covers all members of Part A or Part B with prescription drug coverage. No income verification or physical examinations are required. Health reasons are not a justification for denial. However, over-the-counter medications, life insurance, and high deductibles or premiums may not be covered.

There are four phases of Medicare: the deductible, initial coverage, coverage gap, and catastrophic coverage phases. The deductible phase is where the patient pays 100% of the total drug cost. The initial coverage phase is where the patient typically pays according to the start of their out-of-pocket coverage. The "doughnut hole", also known as the coverage gap, is where the patient pays a defined standard percentage of the total drug cost that is set by the United States Department of Health and Human Services (USDHHS). Lastly, once the catastrophic coverage is reached, USDHHS determines a low percentage that the enrollee is responsible for (ie: five percent).

If patients receive income under a predetermined threshold, healthcare under Medicaid becomes virtually free to the patient. Only low-income people qualify. Under the Affordable Care Act (ACA), standards of minimum coverage include prescription drugs, emergency care, hospitalization, mental health, rehabilitation, preventative services, laboratory tests, childbirth, and pediatric care (Sung, 2016). These comprise the barebones of a health plan. The pros of the Affordable Care Act, also known as ObamaCare, include the regulation that plans must cover at least one drug in every therapeutic category that's stipulated in the United States Pharmacopeia, mental health services up to a set number of therapy visits per year, hospitalization costs up to 20 percent per bill, and preventative and wellness services to drive healthier choices and prevent medical bills (Lalli, 2013). All of these qualifications under that ACA are just the surface; the healthcare system is a massive maze to navigate.

SYSTEM FAILURE

One example of a system failure is the American Opioid Epidemic. Health plans commonly make it harder for patients to fill more expensive, less addictive pain management drugs (Volkow, 2016). They do this by requiring prior authorization, quantity limits, and contingent therapies. These restrictive measures are set on the plan's formulary and essentially drowned prescribers in paperwork. Similarly, health plans limit the duration of therapy on drugs that treat opioid dependence even though it is a chronic condition. This is because the drugs are expensive and health plans don't want to pay for them. Not all of the blame for this epidemic can be placed on health plans. Drug manufactures have much control in lowering drug costs. This epidemic is not due to a lack of knowledge; it's due to a lack of implementation. We as a society created this epidemic. To fix it is not a choice, it's a responsibility.

Another system failure is in the Medicare and Medicaid system. The sheer complexity of the system explains how convoluted it has become. There are numerous players in this system: health plans, government regulations, prescribers, pharmacies, and drug companies. Contracted pharmacy rates, various drug pricing methods, complex manufacture discount calculations, health plan transition policies, benefit phases, out-of-pocket thresholds, incentive fees, administration fees, etc. all contribute to the failures of the healthcare system. And pharmacy insurance is just one segment of the healthcare industry. Lastly, a knowledge term of 10-15 years is unacceptable. There needs to be incentives for drug companies to get new, less toxic drugs to market faster. Health research institutions need permission from their Internal Review Boards (IRBs) to publish their research findings (Esserman, 2016). If researchers needed permission to not publish their data, maybe more drugs would get to market faster.

QUALITY PERFORMANCE SYSTEMS

Big, complex systems need to have quality controls within them. Health institutions, pharmacists, and practitioners need to be kept in check via cross-corporate oversight. Joseph Territo, MD of Kaiser Permanente Medical Group oversees physicians' performance through analyzing clinical data and patient medical records. He believes there's a strong relationship between performance reviews and the Five Stages of Grief (Territo, 2016). At first, when doctors are given bad performance reviews, they start to blame the messenger: "The data isn't right!" And if they find one error, they start to attack the messenger: "*Your* data is inaccurate," or "*Your* data doesn't take into account that my patients are sicker than most." The next stage of grief is anger. This precipitates in the form of hitting "Reply All". Then the bargaining begins, "My patients are sicker," or "My hospital is understaffed." Variation reports can debunk these myths. When showing reports of similar patients and practice settings, the bargaining stops. Depression starts to set-in. The messenger can talk about outcomes rather than process measures. This can cause the recipient to discover success which will cause the depression to subside. Then there's the final stage: acceptance. This can be achieved by making the right thing to do, the easy thing to do. When practitioners are properly monitored, the entire system improves.

IDEAL DELIVERY OF CARE

A Walmart greeter welcomes the customer, engages with him/her, and guides him/her in the right direction. A top health executive for a giant retail chain advocates that this is how health plans should operate (Osbourne, 2016). As health plans sit opportunistically in the middle of patients, doctors, and pharmacists, they're in the perfect position to greet the patient and direct them in the right direction for optimal care. The future of diagnostics is in the form of self-help kiosks (ie: A1C, blood pressure, cholesterol, etc.). Patients want support in navigating the vast healthcare system of today. They want a concierge to help them go to in-network facilities, understand benefit changes, and help them save money. The current healthcare delivery system needs to be flipped on its head. Right now patients fight and get frustrated as they navigate the system. Reverse engineering the system could improve the patient's experience.

Telehealth is another innovation that aids in care delivery. Tuckson believes telehealth will provide tons of value to the healthcare system (Tuckson, 2016). Unlike Osbourne, Tuckson believes telehealth is the concept that is positioned in the best spot in the health system to deliver the optimal value. However, there are some existing barriers in the telehealth industry like a lack of policy, too much regulation, and too much liability. Performance measurement and reimbursement based on telehealth is also non-existent. Creative ways, whether old-fashioned or technical, can greatly improve the delivery of care to patients.

Electronic Health Record

There are potential issues with doctors using EMRs to drive clinical decisions. If all patient data is stored in an EMR, theoretically, that would be the best source of data for the doctor to make clinical decisions. There are lots of medical professionals that often work on the same EMR. This creates room for error as most information updates to

EMRs is manual. Also, if a network has intermittent connectivity, it can delay the time that an end user receives the data. Lastly, if a doctor simply stops using the EMR and goes back to paper charts or other documentation methods, this also creates a great risk. Clinical reasoning based on an EMR is solely based on the assumption that the information the record contains is correct. If an EMR is outdated or contains false data, this can lead to dangerous, inaccurate clinical decisions.

One must understand the procedural and conceptual constructs of mental models in order to translate them into physical, systemic models. Mental models are usually used without conscious awareness (Shortliffe & Cimino, 2013). For example, more experienced system users may be able to use the system flawlessly without really "thinking" about it, whereas an inexperienced user may have to really consciously think about their actions. In order to translate mental models into physical system to be ultimately programmed into artificial intelligence, one must be consciously aware of their thought processes and actions and be able to put them into procedures that can be programmed.

COMPUTERS AND THE MEDICAL PRACTICE

Computers have the ability to support physicians in making clinical decisions and diagnoses while keeping appropriate documentation and audit trails. Previously, computers have made these processes cumbersome. They resulted in lots of time-consuming, manual entry that didn't help the physician come to a conclusion they wouldn't have without the computer (Shortliffe & Cimino, 2013). Some possible ways to make the systems easier are:

1. Designing systems so clerical staff can do all of the data entry and management as currently doctors still use pen and paper for administrative staff to transcribe.
2. Have medical devices that take a measure and feed it into the electronic medical chart. Clinical cell counters, ECG, blood pressure, scales, and temperature machines can directly feed into the computer.
3. Patients can directly enter information into their own chart. Through decision trees and questionnaires with branching logic, the computer can take the responses and convert them to a format that can be entered into the patient chart.
4. A point-and-select approach can also be used. Devices like touch screens, light pens, and PDAs that use wireless networks can allow physicians to access and update patients' charts through mobile connectivity.

The first factor that helps computers assimilate into the medical practice is the new development of computer hardware and software. The size and cost of new devices have decreased, while the amount of storage has increased (Shortliffe & Cimino, 2013). The capabilities and pricing competition have increased too which has led to wider availability and application in the medical field. The second factor is a gradual increase in the number of employees that have been trained in both a health profession and in biomedical informatics. Cross-training is creating more professionals that understand both medical and computer science. Doctors are learning informatics. Computer programmers are learning medical concepts. This cross-training is allowing for better computer systems to be released.

The third factor is changes in healthcare financing which controls increased costs. The newer technologies that are replacing the older technologies are less expensive and produce better diagnostic results. Accuracy, precision, and timing is greatly improved with these new technologies (Shortliffe & Cimino, 2013). One example of this technology is Magnetic Resonance Imaging (MRI) which is used to diagram cross-sectional slices of the body. Previously the measuring of biometrics has been done manually. Now it can be done electronically via handheld devices (ie: blood pressure, temperature, oxygen levels, etc.). Systems need to be cost-effective and deliver patient care cost-effectively too. There's a fine balance between the cost of technology and the value of the patient care that it provides.

An integrated environment for managing medical information would include connecting systems of patient records, clinical trial data, academic research, medical databases, claim and eligibility systems, and nonclinical data. Having all of these types of information in one spot for practitioners to access is extremely powerful and can greatly improve the quality of patient care (Shortliffe & Cimino, 2013). A few ways that system integration could revolutionize the medical practice are improved care due to a continuous flow of patient records, machine learning support in clinical decision trees, and decrease in malpractice if automation is maintained and accurate. Practitioners could see medication adherence in claim data, insurance coverage in eligibility systems, and they could obtain the latest study data for cutting-edge treatment in one place. This would allow practitioners to examine and treat the whole patient.

Biomedical Information Standards

The standardization of biomedical informatics is important because there are many different software platforms, vendor organizations, and governmental regulations that all intertwine. This demonstrates the importance of having standardized qualifiers so that all of these systems have a common denominator and can transfer information between them. Specifically, a solution must determine a way to grant identifiers to facilities and organizations in order to maintain databases and authorize access to such information (Shortliffe & Cimino, 2013). Some of these qualifiers include National Provider IDs, Drug Enforcement Agency numbers, Payor IDs, Employer Identifiers, and member IDs. With all of these qualifiers and identification numbers, systems need a way to store data and present them to clinical users, send warnings about DDIs, recommend dosage changes, and track patient's outcomes. Standards help with the need for agreed upon definitions, qualifiers, and application-specific levels of granularity in the data.

There are lots of organizations, systems, and pieces of data that comprise the Health Information Exchange (HIE). There are three types of standards in HIE: transaction standards, semantic standards, and process standards ("HIE inPractice: Foundation Series", 2013). There is a need to have another transaction standard. The current standards outline the fields and taxonomy of data that gets transferred; however, depending on the destination of the data, the organization and order of the fields are changed. There needs to be a standard that organizes the fields in one order regardless of the destination. All systems need to be able to accept the same organization of data. This would help source systems not have to recompile and reorganize data before communicating with other systems.

SYSTEM COMPLEXITY AND DIFFICULTY OF STANDARDIZATION

Corporations have various acronyms that they use. Even if they're in the same industry, ie: Medicare Part D, they often use different acronyms to reference the exact same thing. For example, one company might say "Patient Residence Code (PRC)" and another company might say "Patient Location Code (PLC)". Even between hospitals this occurs. Sometimes different abbreviations for units differ. For example, one hospital might have 3 intensive care units: NICU (neonatal), PICU (pediatric), and SICU (severe/adults). While smaller hospitals may only have 2 intensive care units: one unit for patients age 0-17 and one unit for patients over the age of 17.

Three challenges with creating standardized medical terminology are variances in organizational structures, information system capabilities, and the reporting formats requested by regulatory bodies. Different organizational structures can cause different terminology to be used. Rural hospitals may be smaller, have fewer medical units, and be delayed in receiving updated regulatory guidance. Varying information system capabilities can also negatively impact the creation of standardized medical terminology. Lastly, depending on the agency a hospital reports to, the agency often requests different naming and reporting formats (ie: CMS, NCQA, FDA, NIH, etc.). Coding and naming schemes vary greatly between medical institutions and is highly dependent on organizational structures, information systems, and regulatory bodies.

Medical professionals are trained to have a questioning attitude. They are also initially trained in a variety of settings where they can see the lack of standardized terminology. Typically, anatomy terminology is standardized via Latin terms and English abbreviations. This is the most important. All of the other reporting, coding, and slang terms are usually not standardized but can be easily

Justin DeCleene MBA, MIS, PBMCT, CPhT

learned overtime. The standardization of medical terms is needed if computers will be used to automate clinical decisions. It's easier to train computers to operate on a standardized terminology rather than add an additional layer of logic to convert between different terminologies between different institutions.

Disruption Caused by eHealth

The largest potential of Biomedical Informatics is that it can be used to detect and prevent errors (Shortliffe & Cimino, 2013). It may seem like a simple task, but when terabytes of data is involved, coupled by numerous source systems, and dynamic government regulations, it can be a challenge. This complex task is met with great reward. Detection of fraud and the prevention of ethical misconduct are just a few large accomplishments that can be achieved.

On the surface, improving technology always seems like a good idea, and usually it is. When it comes to health-care, the more that technology can intervene, the less potential for error. From providing quality information fast to having robots perform surgeries, any complexity of technology can prove beneficial in patient care. Some critics believe that with increased technology, people could lose their jobs. That's not always the case. People are needed to create and maintain technology. Also, there are many instances where technology can do a job, but currently, people still do the job. We are far away from robots conducting clinical trials. Although machine learning is

142

becoming more "human-like", it'll be a longtime before robots will single-handedly do anything. There will always be a need for human intervention.

CONCLUSION

The current healthcare system is unsustainable in terms of affordability, quality, accessibility, and personalization. There are three broad tasks that can improve the current system: expand choice, improve affordability and quality, and speed up the conversion of volume to value. Value is important in any business model (Osterwalder, Pigneur, & Clark, 2010). It's the "difference between what a customer gets from a product, and what he or she has to give in order to get it" ("What is value?", 2017). The way a customer perceives value closely resembles Maslow's hierarchy of needs in that they hold physiological and safety needs at the utmost importance (Almquist, Senior, & Bloch, 2016). Organizations that are focused on their customers and deliver value will succeed in the dynamic, ever-changing healthcare system. Let's challenge the big systems that say we have a certain disease. Let's rise up and challenge the diagnoses that we receive. I'm not saying that we should challenge logic. Let's challenge the response that the current system gives us and respond with a questioning attitude.

Book 3: Internet of Things

13

Technological Shifts

"I believe in the sun even when it rains"

– Anne Frank

The ability of a business to compete both globally and locally increasingly rely on its ability to expand its market share in the digital realm, as well as maintaining critical infrastructure. Many businesses have created information technology (IT) infrastructure and improved the way its staff complete their work. Unfortunately, a lack of understanding of the social, ethical, and security concerns that come with the implementation of information technology affects many businesses today. Technological development in global markets are influenced by an increased pace of development, labor productivity, and competition (Flynn, 2015).

SYSTEMS ANALYSIS

Organizations today use a multitude of different platforms. It's important to consider how different platforms will transfer information between each other. Resources needed to implement and maintain the system need to be planned out to ensure smooth deployment. Lastly, if critical information is not available or the end-user doesn't understand it, the new system will not be beneficial. It's important to keep in mind that a computer will not always transform a poorly organized process into smoothly operating one. There is no point in automating a defective system.

When evaluating any information system, it's important to consider the need of the system. Typically the need is to solve for an inadequacy or inefficiency. The motivation for that need typically surrounds some kind of improvement or lowering of cost. The problem must be defined first before a solution can be evaluated. When evaluating software, it's very important to consider deployment, support, usability, and pricing. It's becoming more common to have integrated software (one software solution for all needs), but there's still a lot of companies that utilize many vendors, and therefore many different pieces of software. These different pieces of software usually "talk" via a web service. In these instances, it's even more vital to conduct system evaluations to plan out compatibility.

System Error or Design Error?

There are lots of failures that can occur in the design alone which can cause system failures. GUI design is very important as it is how the end-user communicates with the system. If the end-user can't figure out how to use the system, then the system is not valuable, and in turn, usually fails during implementation. There's lots of things that designers can do with labeling and describing that can help inform the end-user how to use the system. Sometimes the sheer order and placement of elements can aid in getting the user to understand how to use the system.

Increasing and Unavoidable System Complexity

As companies grow and expand, they acquire and merge with information systems. Each time an additional system gets added or a system's capabilities expand, the complexities and intricacies subsequently increase. Samuel Arbesman believes that system complexity is not a good or bad thing, but rather an inevitable thing (Lucky, 2017). He believes that everything done in the technological realm usually diverts us from elegance and understandability, and towards complexity and unexpectedness. This is illustrated by two important factors: accretion and interconnection. Accretion occurs when newer, larger systems are added to older, smaller systems. This is a common business practice where organizations have a system issue, and instead of fixing the system, they add another system on top of the defective one. It's more common that a system is so complex that no one individual can fully understand it. Complexity does not need to be a scary thing; it's to be expected.

SOCIAL MEDIA AND VIRTUAL COLLABORATION

Social change varies over time. Technological development is related to modernization which is in turn a process of social development. Societies move from one set of economic, political and social arrangements to another (Mandel & Howson, 2015). An issue with social change in any setting is how to see and understand it. One layer of the equation relates to the underlying structure of society and its social institutions. Other factors are how variations can be measured and to what degree of continuity currently persists (Giddens, 1997).

One of the most prominent changes in the way individuals interact with one another is through social media. More events and discussions are held on social media than ever before. This leads many businesses to capitalize on the prospect of highly visible and effective advertising. Employers are therefore relying on social media websites like Facebook and LinkedIn to assess potential employees. Likewise, employees use websites such as Glassdoor to determine salary ranges, interview questions, and employment benefits that companies offer to their employees.

There has been a paradigm shift in the way job seekers look to fill roles and how employers judge these potential employees as a cultural and technical fit for employment. Some companies have replaced the role of the first interview with a thorough online search of social media sites. Employers look for warning signs such as drugs, alcohol, or negative comments about their previous employers (Stoughton, Thompson, & Meade, 2013). Every once in a while employees can be hired or fired due to behavior on social media. Employees that post hurtful, racist, sexist, and threatening posts quickly find themselves out of a job. Some businesses are also finding success at using social media sites to promote business-to-business (B2B) interactions. Social media can increase collaboration between partners and customers, while also offering employees and managers a place to openly and actively discuss ideas. Common examples of social media being used in businesses are providing feedback on policy changes, discussing upcoming laws or regulations, and celebrating employee birthdays (Jussila, Kärkkäinen, & Aramo-Immonen, 2014).

While social media in the business environment does have many benefits, it also may come with a price. Social media in businesses is still a novel concept which is why there are few studies done on the social implications of social media in the workplace. The average user is bombarded with social media and digital messaging which can cause work efficiency to decline. Examples of this are employees skipping important company blog posts or ignoring emails and messages due to the sheer number received and the size. The requirement of accessing and maintaining multiple platforms of redundant communication wastes both time and money (Lee, Son, & Kim, 2015). Another large social issue that has arisen in the modern workplace is the ability to telecommute. With the ability to use virtual private networks, social media, and mobile conferencing systems, working from home has never been easier; however, the efficiency of allowing employees to telecommute is up for debate (Allen, Golden, & Shockley, 2015).

SOCIETAL IMPLICATIONS

The advancement of technology is due to people that are experts in areas of Science, Technology, Engineering, and Math (STEM). In the beginning of the 21st century there was a major shortage of STEM students compared to the number of vacant STEM career positions. However, with all the focus on STEM education, Science and Technology Studies (STS) took a backseat which led to a lack of studying the societal implications of technology. Scientists usually distance themselves from social implications, but the industry is undergoing a shift from "value neutral" to "value driven". Innovation for the sake of innovation is meaningless. Jasanoff says technology can never be neutral because it's always informed by a desired future that doesn't come from the technology itself, but from the societal ideals of what "good" is (Hassler, 2016). We construct ideas of goodness, then innovation and discovery follow that trajectory.

Trust and Ethics

Ethical issues arise not only in a traditional office environment, but in a nontraditional IT setting as well. Although it's not as much of an issue as it was 10 years ago, access can be a large issue when offering services online. Not all individuals have access to devices connected to the Internet, especially those in high risk groups that these services target (Sampson, 2014). These services must carefully balance how their collaboration and communication systems are accessed. For example, if a service is only offered after a digital copy of a current resume is created using a resume builder app, many in those high risks groups would not be able to use such a service. Many public and private services have shifted their billing services to an online platform, which sometimes offers benefits to those that enroll in online services that others cannot use. Even marginal cost reductions, such as not needing to buy stamps and envelopes, can have a substantial impact on those with fixed incomes.

The technological advances in payment systems have made cash all but obsolete in most cases. It is much easier for an individual to call and pay for a bill via a credit card than mail in a check. In many instances, physically going to a location and paying cash is impossible. Billing can be outsourced to another company entirely out of the payee's geographical location. As businesses continue to move away from physical currency and digital services, people without access to these things are left in the dust.

Trust is comprised of ability, integrity, and benevolence (Benamati, Fuller, Serva, & Baroudi, 2010). Ability is that of the organization to provide the service or products that they say they are going to. Integrity is the capacity that the company has to keep their promises. Benevolence is the ability of the company to express to the consumer in the online medium that they are competent and predictable. There have been numerous studies showing that consumers who trust businesses and think they are ethical, are more likely to purchase from that company (Dirks et al, 2011; Bhattacherjee, 2002; Koyuncu & Lien, 2003). Trust is extremely important for e-commerce as it can combat consumer's concerns and doubts (Sharma & Lijuan, 2014). A new concept has been created as a result of this phenomenon: e-loyalty.

E-loyalty is the intention to repurchase from the same website (Chiu, Lin, Sun, & Hsu, 2009). Trust plays a critical role in combating consumer's fear and uncertainty when conducting business via e-commerce channels. Part of gaining the trust of consumers can be done via businesses that use web assurance seals such as VeriSign and TRUSTe. These seals have shown to influence the initial trust of consumers (Sharma & Lijuan, 2014). "Individuality is at the heart of ethics" (Palmer, 2005). The major issue that lies in determining ethical issues in e-commerce is the blurring between the private and public nature of cyber-spaces (Sharma & Lijuan, 2014).

With increased reliance on technology, naturally there are ethical concerns. Machines have been tested with handling court cases, clinical decisions, and directing driving cars ("If Computers Wrote Laws: Decisions Handed Down by Data", 2016). Can machines be trusted enough to handle sensitive information, make life altering decisions, and protect human life? (Goodall, 2016). If machines make a mistake, who is held accountable? As more technology is connected to each other, the dimensions of privacy become more complex.

On the surface, improving technology always seems like a good idea, and usually it is. Some critics believe that with increased technology, people could lose their jobs. That's not always the case. People are needed to create and maintain the technology. Also, there are many instances where technology can do a job, but currently, people still do the job. We are far from robots conducting clinical trials. Although machine learning is becoming more "human-like", it'll be a longtime before robots will single-handedly be able to do anything. There will always be a need for human intervention.

With all of the development of robots and the fact they're becoming so human-like, the technology community is starting to talk about the ethics and rights of robots. Robots are providing life-or-death decisions on court cases and clinical cases. What happens if a robot makes a life-threatening decision in error? Who is responsible? What consequences are faced? Like any other technology, the law is slow to account for the latest technologies. A legal committee in Europe has drafted a report that urges the European Union to adopt rules relevant to all of the latest robot and AI development. The report covers concerns of liability, accountability, and safety (Hassler, 2017). It also presents the need to designate robots as "electronic persons". The community is still divided. One critic argues that "corporations are legal persons, but AIs and chimpanzees aren't" (Hassler, 2017, p. 6). There are still lots of debates about the ethics of robots. The longer it takes for a consensus to be reached, by the time laws are in place, they may not be relevant.

PROS AND CONS OF AUTOMATION

New modes of production rely heavily on information technologies, telecommunications, robotics, and automation. There is a hospital in Baltimore, MD that utilizes Swiss robots to dispense, label, store, package, measure, track, and keep drug inventory. The integration of multiple software systems, machines, and employees can allow for a flawless operation. On the other hand, automation can also negatively impact business operations. While automation may increase the overall efficiency of a business, there are quite a few examples of automation failures. When automation is used to aid in the decision making processes, both complacency and automation biases become an issue (Onnasch, Wickens, & Manzey, 2013). Building upon the previous example, failure of the Baltimore hospital's automation can lead to a myriad of issues if the right safeguards are not in place. A patient's privacy and life could be at risk if the Swiss dispensing robots were to malfunction. While automation is an important aspect of business expansion, it must be done with social, ethical, and security consequences in mind.

Other examples of the effects of new technology on businesses include: strengthened supply chain management, mass customization, and improved customer relationships. Examples of positively impacted organizational opportunities due to transformation into the e-market include:

- Enterprise resource planning (ERP)
- Supply chain optimization
- Utilization of e-markets
- Outsourcing
- Decapitalization of underutilized resources
- Enhanced customer service
- Application of web-based technology tools
- New products and technologies
- New ventures based on corporate knowledge

(Flynn, 2015)

On the other hand, technology has also caused inefficient organization operations. Hardware failures and user error can cause a decrease in the efficiency of a company to do business when they become increasingly reliant on technology. For example, in the year 2000 there was a scarcity of workers that had the technical skills to conduct business in environments of e-commerce (Smith, 2015). This was due to a sudden boom in jobs that required technical expertise and skills that were not held by the majority of employee applicants. An increase in the use of technology in organizations is not strongly correlated to a decrease in jobs.

OFFSHORING AND OUTSOURCING IOT

Businesses are also increasingly relying on office work to be completed in countries that have a lower operating cost. This is known as offshoring. Offshoring is a large issue that tends to divide many individuals, not just the company's stakeholders. This practice completely relies on the ability of offshore employees to function as an onshore employee. Both onshore and offshore employees must be able to collaborate. Unfortunately this raises many social issues for those involved. A social implication of offshoring is the displacement of onshore workers. Depending on the business' country of origin, offshore employees may not be given the same rights and privileges as their onshore counterparts. This can lead to status differences and the potential for abuse in the workplace. If the business is using offshore resources to displace onshore employees, there may be a large amount of resentment and tension in the workplace. This can lead to a failure to collaborate, hit goals, and keep employee turnover low (Levina & Vaast, 2008).

It's usually beneficial for smaller hospitals to outsource IT management to larger hospitals. However, what's to stop the larger hospital from buying out the smaller hospital? In Baltimore, the University of Maryland Medical Center has over 700 beds. They bought up local, smaller hospitals to provide care to patients in the suburbs. It's not that difficult for a massive hospital to buy up smaller ones. Johns Hopkins has done this too. If smaller hospitals outsource their IT, what's next? IT can be a competitive, valuable asset. Outsourcing it may leave the hospital vulnerable to competition and being bought out. Some factors to consider whether or not a medical practice should outsource its information technology functions to a third party are:

- Cost of partnership vs cost of doing services in-house
- Feasibility or access to partnerships
- Technical compatibility of available partnerships
- Outsourcing IT may leave hospitals vulnerable to competition and being bought out

(Reddy, Purao, & Kelly, 2008)

If shared IT platforms are the standard, that can be good because it can lead to an increase of shared information and faster, more accurate clinical decisions. On the other hand, it can be bad because the hacking potential increases when lots of private information is stored in one spot. In addition, one dominant IT platform can decrease competition and raise prices.

APPLICATIONS OF IOT

Adherence to treatment is a major issue in the healthcare field. Technology can help with it. There are many different systems that store medical and nonmedical information. Claim data can be very helpful, but it's reactive in the sense that it's historical and occurs after the medical event. Integrating formulary, cost, benefit, and EHR information can provide real-time data. Patient generated data can also be helpful in gaining real-time data (Canfield & Schelin, 2017). Platforms like Siri and Echo are being tested for interacting with patients like: "Don't go in the fridge again, you're blood sugar is too high", "Remember you have a doctor appointment today", "Did you take your medication?", or "You have a refill due" (Kachnowski, 2017).

C-PAP machines are one of the earliest applications of smart health monitors. The possibilities are endless. A health monitor that is connected to the internet or some form of communication medium can be sent to doctors and aid in patient care. Some of the smart products currently available include wireless pill bottles that track each time the patient opens the bottle and a genetic tracking and reporting tool that is used to analyze a patient's genome (Kachnowski, 2017). These products are a great start, but currently the patient adoption rate of these technologies is rarely greater than 5%. Lots of the wearable technologies that are available today do not collect clinical quality data. If patients aren't adhering to medication or treatment, how can practitioners expect them to adhere to technology? We have the data, we have the platforms, but how do we get the tools to the patients and how do we get the patients to use the tools? Part of the adherence is connected to the user's experience. It's so important that the system is easy to use so that the user likes using it and adherence is increased (Canfield & Schelin, 2017).

Applications of Artificial Intelligence and Augmented Reality

"Internet of Things", "Artificial Intelligence", and "Big Data" may seem like synonymous, buzzwords on the surface, but in reality, their stark differences allude to their similarities. These three concepts are re-writing how we interact, buy and sell, travel, and make things (Brody, 2016). Products such as 3D printers, smart lightbulbs, smart slow cookers, and smart houses are blurring the lines between the realms of virtual and reality. For example, smart slow cookers can be controlled by a smartphone application where the user can set the temperature and cook time and even see the inside of the appliance.

Spending on big data and analytics is not slowing down. IDC Research, Inc. thinks by 2020, revenue from business data and analytics will reach $210 billion. Some of the industries spending the most money on analytics include: banking, healthcare, and insurance ("Business Technology News", 2017). Business Intelligence and Data Analytics are commonly used interchangeably. However, there is a subtle difference. Data Analytics is a broader category that Business Intelligence fits into: Business Intelligence is a type of Data Analytics ("Business Intelligence vs Data Analytics", 2015). Business Intelligence seeks to answer business questions through analytics.

Augmented Reality (AR) seeks to blur the lines between the digital and physical worlds (Pretz, 2016a). The capabilities and applications of AR are vast. People with disabilities could use AR to restore their senses (ie: sight, hearing, touch, etc.) and increase their abilities. A disabled person could jump, see, and travel to places in AR that they couldn't do in real life. This is gaining lots of attention in the medical community. American veterans commonly suffer from post-traumatic stress disorder (PTSD). Dr. Rizzo, owner of an AR startup Bravemind, says that PTSD is "about confronting your past and moving past it" (Popescu, 2017). He believes that AR can be a form of prolonged exposure therapy for treating PTSD. The simple immersion can be used to help treat pain, addiction, phobias, sexual trauma, and Parkinson's.

Critics of AR

Critics of AR voice concerns over privacy, addiction, and ethics. Google Glass failed due to privacy concerns that consumers' activities were being recorded (Pretz, 2016b). Like any other technology, the user can become addicted. Just like online video games, users can become so addicted that they can't tell what's real and what's not. On the other hand, it can improve a person's quality of life by providing a better, alternative, and virtual world that makes them happy. Lastly, there are concerns about enhancing performance. Similar to performance enhancing drugs, AR applications such as implants and prosthetics could give some competitors an unfair advantage (Pretz, 2016b).

MEDICAL COGNITION AND NATURAL LANGUAGE PROCESSING

Generating access to care is especially useful in cancer care. IBM's Watson can be deployed in a rural location and provide cutting-edge technology, information, and recommendations to cancer patients that wouldn't normally have access to oncologists. The ultimate goal of Watson is to leverage compiled data and to "think" new thoughts from that data. It's the next generation of artificial intelligence: cognitive systems. Cognitive Science is the coordination of theory and evidence. The field aims to establish founding principles of related social sciences and applications. Cognitive Science is heavily grounded in philosophy, behavioral psychology, and verifiable observations with the end goal of synthesizing many fields of study and theories with this modern technological framework (Shortliffe & Cimino, 2013).

Medical Cognition is the organization of clinical and scientific knowledge. Information system architectures organize physical memory, while theories usually organize content (Shortliffe & Cimino, 2013). Cognitive psychology has helped dictate constructs and variability of engaging taxonomies for artificial intelligence. The system needs to be able to take in stimuli, adapt to it and interpret it, and output meaningful processed information (Shortliffe & Cimino, 2013). This is also referred to as the represented world and the representing world. Biomedical informatics is the development and use of medical knowledge bases, medical artificial intelligence, or decision support systems to prevent medical errors (Shortliffe & Cimino, 2013).

Natural Language Processing (NLP) has been used in the biomedical and health domains in functions such as information extraction, information retrieval, text generation, user interfaces, and machine translation (Shortliffe, Cimino, 2013). Knowledge forms that are used in NLP include morphology, lexicography, syntax, semantics, and pragmatics (Shortliffe & Cimino, 2013). Morphology is the combination of morphemes (roots, prefixes, suffixes) to produce words. Lexicography is the categorization of lexemes (the words and atomic terms) of the language. Syntax is the structure of the phrases and sentences. Semantics is the meaning or interpretation of words, phrases, and sentences. Pragmatics is how sentences combine to form discourse. The ultimate goal of NLP and AI is being able to collect information, form opinions, adjust opinions and put it all together for a specific purpose ("Cognitive Computing Explained", 2017). Once AI is able to mimic how the human brain works, it will be able to process natural language and have the capability to learn.

Challenges of NLP

Challenges for NLP in the clinical domain occur due to the limited availability of electronic records, manual data entry mistakes, subjective interpretation of notes, and the large number of different clinical domains. Like other domains, there is a lack of standards which further complicates the development of NLP (Shortliffe, Cimino, 2013). Clinical information needs to be interpreted, but that's difficult because of the backend clinical knowledge base that would need to be built. Challenges for NLP in the biological domain typically exist due to the complexity and the lack of standard nomenclature. The ambiguity and multidisciplinary approach of the names make it difficult to create automated processing of the data. There are a large number of biomolecular entities which further complicate NLP in the biological domain. Lastly, the fact that most biological research information is housed in paper abstracts complicates the automated processing of it. Abstracts are free-text and not standardized. That's why it's difficult to conduct NLP in the biological domain.

CONCLUSION

Software is a major piece of the app economy. Software as a Service and Mobility as a Service are frameworks that companies are implementing to help them differentiate from their competitors (Markman, 2016). Uber and Lyft are just two companies that are prospering from Mobility as a Service where the company uses mobility connectivity as a medium to provide their services to customers. Every business is different and will therefore be subjected to different ethical issues. No set of ethical standards will ever exist; therefore, each business will need to adopt its own set of ethical standards. However, addressing key ethical issues that occur in every business model seem to hold true in IT as well. Responsibility, respect, honesty, and fairness need to be considered when expanding a business into the digital realm.

Currently, developers of AR are finding it challenging to be able to incorporate touch, smell, and taste into their technologies. It's important that they're able to do this in order to create a completely immersive world. The ultimate goal of AR is to provide a virtual world that is so real that the user doesn't notice it's not real.

The new paradigm in employee-employer relationships created by social media, telecommuting, and offshoring has resulted in many great opportunities to maximize growth and decrease operating expenses. However, the implications of using these methods to increase business efficiency can come with extensive social ramifications.

When dealing with these new tools it has become clear that the roll out and maintenance of them require careful consideration from management so the business doesn't travel down an unethical and unprofitable road that may have vast unforeseen consequences.

14

Implementation of HIMS in Foreign Countries

OVERVIEW OF DHIS2

DHIS2 is an open-source software that allows a seamless transfer of health information across geographical borders. The software makes it easy for the end-user to generate reports, charts, graphs, and maps in order to accurately communicate data-driven conclusions in real time. There are numerous obstacles when implementing any type of system; however, DHIS2 has an enormous amount of documentation and manuals that aid in the implementation process. As with any system, there are pros and cons. DHIS2 is targeted towards rural, developing countries and improving their healthcare system in regards to the transfer of information. Pros, cons, recommendations, and feasibilities will be explored.

CASE STUDIES

Health Information Management Systems (HIMS) seeks to reduce risk, predict costs, and respond to the medical needs of a population. The wave of the future is to have HIMS support the pharmaceutical industry, comply with government regulations, and increase the responsiveness and effectiveness of the overall healthcare system. Capabilities of HIMS that can support the overall goal are to coordinate, protect, and distribute resources effectively. Previously rural cities are surfacing with mega cities; they are requiring social and cultural changes. The healthcare systems in those cities are no exception. This has sparked a healthcare revolution. Malaria and Tuberculosis are major issues in Pakistan and other rural areas. Tasks of HIMS include: oversight, welfare, laws, and preventative programs (Mashhadi, Hamid, Roshan, & Fawad, 2016). There is a severe problem with the coordination and duplication of HIMS in general.

Sometimes countries implement HIMS in such a way that puts more emphasis on data rather than actions. The entire point of HIMS is the ability to retrieve data to aid in effective decision making and actions. Common challenges that companies face in regards to HIMS include a lack of medical professionals that also have IT skills (Matavire, 2016), a lack of network or computer infrastructure (Mashhadi, Hamid, Roshan, & Fawad, 2016), and poor implementation in general (Bhattacharya, Shahrawat, & Joon, 2012).

INDIA AND AUSTRALIA

Common issues that surround HIMS reporting systems include: no data reported due to a lack of services, a lack of technical skills, HIMS data collection is too extensive, and confusion surrounding deadlines. Countries seek to use HIMS for strengthening health systems and to initiate change in health policies at a local level. India looked to Australia for ideas on how to implement a successful HIMS. Australia has structured their systems in such a way that supports the dissemination of data across all geographical boundaries. They have five major functional databases that house surveillance and emergency information (Tiwari, Kumar, Raj, & Kulkarni, 2016). The purpose of the vast network that Australia has deployed is to link data and provide relevant services to its people.

The author's Tiwari et al (2016) recommend an extensive information system that allows for evidence-based policy making. The standardization of health data is critical to this endeavor (Bhattacharya et al, 2012). It is pertinent that any HIMS provides reliable data. There also needs to be a single portal that integrates all of the information systems. Integration can be easier if the data is standardized. The ultimate goal is to have data in a fixed format and in an easily accessible location. Having a single national health institution can help with these initiatives, in order to eventually get to achieve a non-fragmented, and consistent HIMS. India is noticing that some of these initiatives are actually creating bottlenecks. The bottlenecks that are popping up is just the tip of the iceberg of problems. These operational problems include poor data quality, lack of understanding of data fields, and manual entry issues. Again, data sets need to be standardized and equipment needs to be maintained properly (Bhattacharya et al, 2012; Tiwari et al, 2016).

GHANA

Ghana has a unique HIMS. The Integrated Disease Surveillance and Response (IDSR) system has core and supporting functions at all levels of the nation. Data submissions to the IDSR have been made easier via the implementation of mobile phones (Adokiya, Awoonor-Williams, Beiersmann, & Müller, 2016). Since none of the health facilities had system manuals, technical guidelines, competent supervisors, or good laboratories, the data that was being submitted was poor and untrustworthy. This poor data naturally lead to poor decision making.

Ghana's IDSR is like DHIS2 but it only reports on diseases. It was originally intended to be a comprehensive public health strategy. The ultimate goal of IDSR is to integrate multiple vertical health systems so that it can act as a single source of information. Ghana hopes to integrate IDSR into DHIS2 so that the reporting burden is lessened, data quality is improved, and duplicate efforts are reduced; however, the integration caused some issues. Issues that have risen from the implementation of Ghana's HIMS include: unstable power supplies, poor data collection, a lack of laboratory capacity, and false medical diagnoses. Data transmission issues have been mediated via local, mobile phones and district-level data entry clerks transcribing paper records. Ghana was a recipient of the

AfDB 2013 Award Winner on eHealth ("DHIS2 in Action", 2016). Ghana's DHIS2 system is setup to routinely collect aggregate data every month. District hospitals capture case-based data from inpatient admissions and deaths via ICD-10 codes. Ghana has found that the implementation of DHIS2 has aided in more accurate morbidity and mortality statistics.

In conclusion, there have been many positive initiatives in Ghana's HIMS. Better availability and access to reports have been a result of integrating IDSR with DHIS2 (Adokiya, Awoonor-Williams, Beiersmann, & Müller, 2016). A survey was distributed to health professionals that use DHIS2. The results showed that the majority of staff did not think the integration improved surveillance activities. It also showed that they were not satisfied with the system's performance.

KENYA

Kenya was the first Sub-Sahara African county to implement a 100% online, national HIMS. All of Kenya's district health facilities are connected via mobile internet (ie: USB modems). District Officers from all over Kenya use the Interpretations feature of DHIS2 to share charts and medical interventions to improve healthcare in the country ("DHIS 2 In Action", 2016). On a daily basis, users of DHIS2 are able to send messages and/or requests to support the National Data Officers. A challenge that Kenya is noticing when implementing DHIS2 is that it is not an "end all" solution to accurate healthcare reporting (Karuri, Waiganji, Orwa, & Manya, 2014). Kenya is having difficulties maintaining the system which is causing the disjoints that the system is experiencing today. Kenya is trying to deploy DHIS2 vertically, horizontally, and geographically in efforts of bridging these gaps. DHIS2, like any other system, needs to be monitored and maintained. Kenya needs to add the appropriate infrastructure to effectively support staff and maintain the system.

Socio-technical challenges arise when deploying DHIS in developing, rural countries. This exacerbates the already unpredictable and uncertain environment. There needs to be continued monitoring of how district-level healthcare professionals are reporting data. An outcome of continued monitoring should be that trends in clinical informatics lead to process improvements and new strategies to combat uncertainty. As with the other countries that have implemented DHIS2, Kenya faced some challenges. These challenges could have been addressed in the requirements gathering and the feasibility analysis phases. Internet connectivity, user capacity, and capital should have been addressed in the feasibility analysis and could have resulted in better remediation of these activities.

The goal of any HIMS is to produce quality data that can be used to support evidence-based decision making, and to intervene and improve clinical outcomes. Most of the time, when rural countries implement DHIS2, there is the issue of a lack of access to computers and internet services. Typically, countries will have the district-level facilities fill out paper forms that are then sent to national offices for transcription. Kenya overcame this by deploying mobile devices.

PAKISTAN

Pakistan uses DHIS to measure morbidity and mortality of major diseases along with long-term planning and management of healthcare services. DHIS in Pakistan has a strong presence at the provincial level. However, the employees that interface with DHIS are usually not motivated, not trained, and don't use the data to make decisions (Nawaz, Ali Khan, & Khan, 2015). There is an opportunity to improve the integration of DHIS with other vertical information systems in order to improve the quality of data and ultimately make better data-driven decisions. The capacity of DHIS managers needs to be evaluated. There needs to be an assessment of capacity at the district-level so that the system is supported appropriately at all levels.

The staff members that are involved in reporting statistics through DHIS2 in Pakistan are typically skilled in data collection and aid in the overall process of compiling monthly reports and storing them on computers at the district office. There is an opportunity to get more funding from the government as there is a severe lack of resources, staff, and knowledge banks. District-level employees do not have reporting, analysis, or communication skills causing the majority of data values to be missing.

One of the greatest challenges facing Pakistan's HIMS is getting employees to commit to the utilization and maintenance of the system. The reason for this challenge is the political instability of Pakistan and high staff turnover. Another challenge that Pakistan's HIMS faces is that the country's general healthcare system is highly segmented, uncoordinated, and unintegrated (Nawaz, Khan, & Khan, 2015). There needs to be a health policy in place that addresses all areas of the healthcare system such as DHIS, research, monitoring, and supervision. Training workshops could also combat the high staff turnover. Gaining commitment from HIMS Managers on the implementation of DHIS2 is critical to its success. There needs to be a health policy that addresses all areas of the health system.

There are numerous areas of weakness in Pakistan's implementation of DHIS2. Of course, Pakistan is experiencing the typical struggles that other rural countries experience such as a lack of internet, resources, skilled staff, accountability, and communication (Mashhadi, Hamid, Roshan, & Fawad, 2016). Pakistan has a severe weakness and a system risk due to its fragmented, uncoordinated, and unintegrated healthcare system; hardware is not maintained, there is a lack of governance, and reporting is not being used as intended. If Pakistan's healthcare leaders do not fix these shortfalls, DHIS2 in

Pakistan will be obsolete and worthless shortly after its implementation.

TANZANIA

The first HIMS that Tanzania used was MTUHA. Due to its lack of source code, the program was very rigid and not customizable. Data fields couldn't be moved around and data validation was incompatible. Tanzania also had a prior version of DHIS implemented. DHIS1.3 was housed in Microsoft Access and was coded according to the context of Tanzania's landscape (Kiwanuka, Kimaro, & Senyoni, 2015). Tanzania implemented DHIS2 in 2013. It has made huge improvement efforts which have led to the wide success that their system experiences today. Tanzania integrated their IDSR system into DHIS2 and rolled out weekly reporting via mobile devices. Lastly, Tanzania has also integrated their Pay for Performance system into DHIS2. The flexibility of DHIS2, the skilled users and supervisors, and the highly integrated systems in Tanzania has led to a widely successful healthcare system ("DHIS2 in Action", 2016).

There are lots of health institutions that deal with health reporting in Tanzania. The country should streamline their governing bodies so that healthcare professionals are held more accountable and reporting can be even more accurate. Innovation is initially fueled by its promised benefits; however, it proves difficult when organizational habits are trying to be changed at the same time (Kumar,

Maheshwari, & Kumar, 2002; Williamson, Kaasbøll, Braa, & Sun, 2008). This was evident in transitioning from paper to electronic medical records in Tanzania. The Health Metrics Network tried to aid in this transition in Tanzania and other African countries (Sæbø, Kossi, Titlestad, Tohouri, & Braa, 2011).

One way they effectuated this change is by linking data entry to employee performance reviews. If employees didn't start collecting health data in the approved format, their performance reviews would suffer. Kiwanuka, Kimaro, and Senyoni suggest that DHIS be integrated with vertical health systems so that Tanzania has a pool of resources for training and human resources (2015). These simple actions would speed up this change process.

UGANDA, ZAMBIA, AND LATIN-AMERICA

Uganda

Uganda is another country that is being creative with the customization of DHIS2. They are enhancing the capabilities of the national HIMS. First, it only took an impressive 6 months for Uganda to implement DHIS2. This was largely due to the expansion of mobile internet networks. Secondly, Uganda has used DHIS2 to track mothers and children across a continuum of healthcare to measure key performance indicators on maternal health, and to allow system users at all levels to submit data directly into the database.

Zambia

Zambia deployed DHIS2 in a targeted manner. The country used DHIS2 to support its Malaria Vaccine Initiative. Mobile DHIS2 devices have been used to collect minimum datasets to monitor these trends. The aggregate data is then sent to the National Malaria Control Center in Zambia via a Java national DHIS2 instance ("DHIS2 in Action", 2016). The National Malaria Control Center did a good job of meeting the needs of the system at the local level.

Latin-America

In general, the region of Latin America has many countries that are currently in progress of adopting DHIS2. The region has DHIS2 Academy Workshops, research networks, and pilot studies to support implementation efforts. DHIS2 developers have started joint workshops in Oslo, Norway; Spain; and Latin America. Pilot studies were started in Colombia, Mexico, and Paraguay. All of these workshops and studies have contributed to the rapid dissemination of the DHIS2 program.

ZIMBABWE

Zimbabwe's HIMS started out strong. Their national health institutions recruited, hired, and trained lots of stakeholders. They introduced HIMS courses to polytechnic schools in the area to improve the abilities of students to handle massive sets of data. In theory, this is a great initiative; however, it led to a period of hyperinflation in the job market which caused skilled workers to emigrate from Zimbabwe. This was detrimental to Zimbabwe's healthcare system.

A pain point in Zimbabwe's DHIS2 implementation is that it is heavily dependent on the support of private donors. It is safe to assume it is therefore not supported by the government or political system and its longevity is only as long as its donors support it. The national HIMS in Zimbabwe is generally weak. Private donations usually fund vertical systems. DHIS2 easily integrates many kinds of diverse systems. It is good that donors are supporting DHIS2. Hopefully DHIS2 will prove to be the sustainable, integrated solution that the country of Zimbabwe needs.

Before Zimbabwe implemented DHIS2, they used DHIS 1.4. DHIS 1.4 was housed in Microsoft Access at the district, provincial, and national levels. Data clerks, if they had access to computers, would use custom forms for data entry. For clerks that did not have access to computers, they recorded data on paper and forwarded it to a district or national office for data transcription. The database was stored offline. If the office was closed, or if staff was unavailable, the data was inaccessible. If the Ministry of Health and Child Care (MOHCC) was on a site visit traveling, they would take the desktop that hosted the national database. DHIS2 allowed for greater mobility. The implementation of DHIS2 in Zimbabwe was extremely rapid. This was partly due to the support from the developers of DHIS2 in Oslo, Norway. The patient tracker and GIS modules were pre-built which also aided the rapid integration.

SYSTEM CRITIQUE

Pros of DHIS2

DHIS2 does a fantastic job of creating a logical GUI. The majority of the button names are indicative of what their function is. Other names are less descriptive but their function can be found in the copious amounts of software literature. Numerous features mimic Microsoft Excel which allows the training curve to be minimal if the end-user is familiar with Excel. Graphs, pivot tables, dashboards, and intensity maps can be generated easily via the logical flow of the GUI.

For more technically inclined users, DHIS2 allows for a variety of programming platforms (ie: SQL, Eclipse, PHP, JAVA). The GUI of DHIS2 utilizes an application layout. The GIS app allows for the generation of intensity maps. The Data Visualizer app allows for the generation of tables and graphs. In the end, DHIS can export data in numerous formats (ie: PDF, XLS, CSV, JSON, XML, SQL, JRXML). In addition to export formats, there are multiple ways of viewing data analytics within the program browser. The most basic reports are built via pivot tables, but allow for more styling and formatting options than Excel. Reports can be repeatedly generated via a single-click and can be downloaded as a PDF. Dashboards can be customized to show the end-user only the data that they want to see in real-time. Four customized charts, favorite reports, tables, and map views can be configured in the dashboard (DHIS 2 End User Manual, 2016). The Data Visualizer App can display numerous indicators and data elements at the same time and in a meaningful way. Charts and reports generated from this app can be added to a personal dashboard or downloaded as an image file or a PDF.

Another type of report that can be generated from DHIS2 is Organization Distribution Reports. They show the number and type of health facilities that are in any area within any hierarchy of the healthcare system. These Organization Distribution Reports can display the information in tables, charts, PDFs, Excel, and CSV files. For internal reporting audits, there is a feature that DHIS2 has to communicate the amount of data being entered into the system. The Reporting Rate Summary can help administrators and executives determine if the system is being utilized frequently. Granted this only alludes to the quantity and not the quality of the data being entered, but it provides metrics that can be used to communicate a message. Lastly, the GIS App can allow the end-user to view thematic maps, hierarchies, and organizational units.

DHIS2 is an open-source software, meaning it can be easily integrated with other systems. Depending on the countries' current healthcare information system, it may be beneficial for the country to house all healthcare data in DHIS2. Ghana and Tanzania have integrated their vaccine monitoring system with DHIS2 in order to enhance the capabilities of their current system (Adokiya, Awoonor-Williams, Beiersmann, & Müller, 2016; Kiwanuka, Kimaro, & Senyoni, 2015). Having the two systems integrated decreased reporting errors and system transfer issues. The flexibility of DHIS2 is a great asset to countries.

Cons of DHIS2

The ease of navigation through a program's Graphic User Interface (GUI) is crucial to the success of the software's adoption. Being able to self-learn and navigate the GUI on one's own without referring to a manual is important for a company to implement the software in a timely manner. Most of DHIS2's buttons are easy to understand and described the function of the button; however, some button names are not that logical. For example, buttons with names such as "Column", "Row", and "Indicator" are rather obvious. On the other hand, buttons with names such as "User sub-x2-units" may not be as obvious. The simple renaming of some buttons can greatly benefit the implementation of the system.

In addition to the naming of the buttons, the patient profile GUI is not that comprehensive. There are numerous key patient identification fields that are missing (ie: patient ID, date of birth, city, etc.). There is no way to determine if there is duplicate patient data entered into the system. In order to intake a complete patient medical history, it's important that all of the key metrics are able to be entered into the system and generated on reports. DHIS2 should add more input fields so that the decisions of health professionals can be more targeted and specific.

The purpose of DHIS2 is to "help governments in developing countries and health organizations manage their operations more effectively, monitor processes, and improve communication" ("DHIS2 in Action", 2016). There is a clear need in the software industry to have a strong system that can handle medical records and provide analytics on geographical information. Data charting that overlay geographical maps can help communicate important stories about the data. This type of information has the most notable application in epidemiology. Health Geographical Analytics is something that DHIS2 excels at; however, DHIS2 is so focused on that niche type of analytics that it neglects some basic charting functions.

Lastly, the pivot tables in DHIS2 are a bit clunky and the types of graphs available are limited. In Microsoft Excel it is clear where to drop data fields and where they will be located in the pivot table. In DHIS2, the Data Visualizer is not logical as to where the data fields will be located in the pivot. DHIS2 has done a great job at geographical mapping. Now it needs to shift focus on developing the neglected, non-geographical analytic tools.

MOBILITY IN FOREIGN COUNTRIES

DHIS2 mobile reporting allows healthcare professionals to collect, transmit, and analyze data in a timely manner in order to accurately monitor and respond to public healthcare outbreaks ("DHIS2 in Action", 2016). DHIS2 mobile reporting is technically feasible and sustainable. It is customizable to meet the needs of the country at the local level. The technology utilizes cheap mobile phones with prepaid SIM cards to send data to the DHIS2 server; however, deploying HIMS in foreign countries is complex and difficult. The lack of internet connectivity, computer hardware, and access to medicine directly impacts the implementation of HIMS. In addition, the high prevalence of poverty and disease work against positive health outcomes. Nyella and Kimaro believe that all of this can be remediated via managing the flow of geographical boundaries and standardizing data models (2016). They recommend that community DHIS authorities need to circulate devices and resources to accommodate the diverse needs of data.

CONCLUSION

DHIS2 is an open source electronic health record system used in developing countries. Some general factors that can contribute positively or negatively to the implementation of healthcare technology include: human resource capacities, the perception of the new technology, and employees' commitment to supporting and maintaining the system (Kiwanuka, Kimaro, & Senyoni, 2015). DHIS2 is a highly flexible, easy to implement, and cost-effective healthcare reporting solution. Applications of the software include the monitoring and rationing of medical supplies, the analysis of population statistics and diseases, and the integration of a Pay-Per-Performance solution. DHIS2 is a beneficial healthcare analytics solution that can be useful in any country.

15

Privacy, Security, and Information Sharing

Technological advances have allowed Internet speeds to increase at an unprecedented rate. The availability and application of the Internet have caused an increase in the opportunity to commit computer crimes (Zaharia, Zaharia, Tudorescu, & Zaharia, 2010). Webpages are constantly monitoring visitor traffic in the background regardless of whether or not the visitor gives consent (Reconciling E-Commerce and Privacy, 1998). Some privacy issues that occur online are: domain name squatting, hijacking of web sites, piracy, defamation, theft of copyright material, and blackmail (Lawrence, Culjak, & Lawrence, 2003).

HIGH RISK SETTINGS

Data Sharing in Healthcare

There are incentives to implement information exchange systems but there are no incentives that actually make vendors want to implement them. In fact, it's beneficial for them not to. There are lots of regulations around privacy and medical information. Usually patients need to sign multiple waivers just to allow insurance companies to share medical information with their own third-party vendors. From a vendor perspective, there is no incentive to create these exchange systems because they would have to have an open or compatible platform which would cause it not to be proprietary and therefore not profitable. There should be some kind of feasible incentive solution that would make vendors want to collaborate while maintaining profits at the same time. Sadly enough, this scenario happens in the healthcare industry too often.

Facial Images

It is rare nowadays that a consumer can find a device without a camera in it. Sixty-five percent of Americans are taking selfies on smartphone cameras, and databases that collect our visages are rapidly expanding (Jain & Kofman, 2017). It is highly likely that the average person has a picture of their face taken once a day without them knowing. There is always a privacy concern that exists if one is in front of electronics, especially social media. Something as seemingly innocent as police body cameras that were implemented to hold officers accountable for their actions, are being used for facial recognition technology. A face picture can be taken from a body camera, uploaded to multiple databases, and tagged for recognition later.

Police have even taken a picture for one reason and placed it in an unrelated database. The breach of privacy is hidden and surprisingly intertwined with everyday devices.

Partnerships

Due to the increasingly minute distinction between virtual and physical reality, it is getting difficult to determine if privacy concerns in e-commerce are qualitatively or quantitatively different than those in physical reality (Bennett, 2001). The structure of a business itself can lead to privacy issues. For example, the more companies that are involved, the more possible areas where information can leak out (Bennett, 2001). A health insurance company is a good example that utilizes a vendor, a medical center partnership, and may merge with other insurance companies. All of these parties are more points where information can leak out to people that shouldn't have protected health information. It is important for the organization to secure these access points in order to protect customers from intruders.

Volunteering Information and Robot Calls

In addition to user traffic, businesses can also collect information directly from the user. For example, online forms collect information that the user enters. Companies may offer incentives such as giveaways or raffles in order to get the user to give up this information (Reconciling E-Commerce and Privacy, 1998). Just because users enter in the information, does not make it right for companies to sell it; that's both a privacy and ethical issue. Robot calling is also covered under privacy regulations and rules. Just because a phone number is on a robot calling list does not equate to consent from the recipient of the phone call. Robot callers are liable for phone numbers that have been reassigned. Meaning that if a number was reassigned, the caller is responsible for getting consent from the new owner of that number. There is however one loophole as an initial call needs to take place in order to establish the consent from the new owner of the phone number (Internet Law Regulatory and Litigation Matters, 2015).

Phishing

Phishing is another form of privacy breach. It is an attack where the attacker poses as a company and collects financial information from the victim. There are two new forms of phishing that have emerged recently: spear phishing and Business Email Compromise (BEC). Spear phishing occurs when a legitimate looking email is sent to the victim. The victim opens the email and/or file which steals personal information. The most common file type involved in these phishing attacks is Rich Text Format (RTF). Employees should be instructed not to open these files from unknown senders (Caldwell, 2013). An example of an attack like this occurred May 2015 where 200,000 social security numbers from the IRS data warehouse were leaked (Dave, 2015). Because of this, dispute papers had to be filed if someone did not receive their tax return. Also, Identity Protection numbers were created as an extra level of security. Lastly, credit freezes were put in place to prevent new accounts from being opened under a fraudulent social security number.

Business Email Compromise (BEC) is another form of phishing. The Federal Bureau of Investigation published the following statistics regarding BECs from October 2013 to August 2015:

	Victims	Dollars
US	7,066	$747,659,840.63
Non-US	1,113	$51,238,118.62
Total	8,179	$798,897,959.25

(Business Email Compromise, 2015)

Eighty-six percent of all BECs occur in the United States. This demonstrates the prevalence of attacks. If an attack occurs on a company, it is important that the company understands how the attack happened and what can be done to prevent it in the future.

OTHER PRIVACY BREACHES

- August 24, 2000: Microsoft is made aware of expired Hotmail accounts retaining the Instant Messenger buddy lists for the next account owner to access.

- September 6, 2000: IKEA's online catalog website accidentally published over 10,000 customer's financial information online.
- October 12, 2000: Buy.com's website exposed customer's personal information online for those who return products back to the company.
- January 3, 2001: AT&T's website exposed thousands of small businesses financial information online.
- January 22, 2001: Travelocity exposed thousands of customers billing information online.

(Bennett, 2001)

A creepy story regarding privacy breaches came out in the Forbes magazine on February 16th, 2012 ("How Target Figured out a Teen Girl Was Pregnant before Her Father Did", 2012). A man's daughter kept receiving coupons in the mail addressed to her for baby stuff. She was still in high school. Her dad was furious. Turns out, she was pregnant. Target tracks consumer purchases and assigns pregnancy scores to them. Based on the scores, specialized coupon books are sent to specific customers. When people began expressing their dissatisfaction with this practice, Target started putting lawn mower ads next to baby diapers so the ads didn't appear so targeted. Turns out, consumers were more likely to use the coupons if they didn't think they were getting spied on. This is just one example of the depth of information a company can collect about its customers.

INTERNET REGULATION

Who owns the internet? Perhaps the people do as they are the ones generating the content. Perhaps it's the government of various countries as they have the power to regulate what is able to be published. Countries are adopting different approaches of regulating the internet depending upon their societal and cultural values (Lawrence, Culjak, & Lawrence, 2003). The United States has the most sophisticated internet regulations. The laws are vague which allows loopholes and debates to ensue about what is actually allowed on the internet. France is thinking about implementing manual monitoring of the internet. If they do this, they would join other countries in what is known as the Communist bloc.

Singapore utilizes a blacklist that maintains a list of sites that citizens are not allowed to access. There are about 100 sites, mostly pornographic, that are on the list. Singapore Broadcasting Authority regulates the blacklist. Some classes of content are automatically authorized as long as established practices are followed. At one point China went as far as requiring Internet users to register with the police. Germany has a new, unique law that outlines the legal liabilities of Internet Service Providers (ISPs) when illegal material passes through them (Ang, 2015). The variance in Internet laws across different countries demonstrate the difference in e-commerce content and operations that need to be personalized to each country's regulations.

SECURITY METHODS

Computer hackers are finding many different ways to not be detected by security software including hiding pieces of code that would be flagged as an attack. Security solutions are getting just as smart ("Security Terms Unlocked", 2017). Behavior-based monitoring looks at a given program and the overall network to see how the performance changes over time. Cloud access security brokers apply security policies to the system. Machine learning technologies get smarter overtime by analyzing the patterns and behavior of the computer. User behavior analytics (UBA) and user and entity behavior analytics (UEBA) seek to identify inside threats by looking at the user's behavior. Like most methods, one is not viable for all settings.

Protection in the Cloud

Cloud computing is still an ambiguous buzzword. Each major technology company defines it a little differently (Luqmani, 2014). NIST defines cloud computing as a model for enabling convenient, on-demand network access to a shared pool of computing resources. IBM views cloud computing as cost-efficient model for distributing processes, applications and services while simplifying IT management simpler and increasing business responsiveness. Microsoft defines cloud computing as a method of distributing and scaling services on shared hardware.

Cloud security is an issue not only for consumers, but also for businesses. Companies hold highly classified information on their cloud servers. Consumers need to be assured that their information is safe with the company they do business with. Likewise, companies need to ensure their proprietary material is safe on their servers because if it gets compromised, the company's vitality is on the line. E-Businesses are getting more and more involved in legal and security incidents (Fusilier & Penrod, 2009). The average cost per incident is $6.65 million (Meisner, 2009). Trust is not only a component of ethics, but also a component of security and fraud in relation to e-commerce. Characteristics of an appropriate, effective legal environment for businesses conducting transactions in e-commerce should:

- protect consumers and intellectual property rights
- foster digital security enablers, such as authentication of online transactions
- allow new businesses to register quickly and easily (Fusilier & Penrod, 2009)

The Federal Trade Commission published that credit card fraud makes up 25% of all reported fraud (Parayitam, Desai, & Desai, 2008). Although companies spend a lot of time and money in communicating how they're protecting the customer from security breaches, there are still many breaches occurring. This may cause one to question whether or not a company is actually implementing the security measures they communicate to their customers.

Data Minimization

Data Minimization is gaining popularity in the literature. It is a technique that is employed to protect the privacy and information of consumers by having companies only hold onto the information about consumers that they absolutely need. Companies hold terabytes of information in their databases. Data minimization puts the nature of the information into question. Are companies holding more information about their customers than they actually need? Do companies have a purpose for every piece of information about their customers that they save? If companies are holding more information than what they utilize on a daily basis to meet the needs of their consumers, there's high potential for a security breach (Brown, 2016). If the company's database gets attacked, all of the information can go into the hands of the wrong people. If data minimization is employed, in the event of a security breach, less information gets in the wrong hands. It has been estimated that a loss of $1 billion in 2006 e-commerce was sustained due to customers' concerns of online security (Parayitam, Desai, & Desai, 2008). It is of monetary value for companies to ensure their customers that shopping on their website is safe.

Payment Methods

Apple Pay has revolutionized the way that people pay. Secure Electronic Transaction (SET), the technology that Apple Pay uses, may have some vulnerabilities.

Eventually fraudsters will find ways to tap into this wireless signal and intercept the information from the phone before it reaches the point of sale (POS) system (Lawrence, Culjak, & Lawrence, 2003). Although lines between social and privacy issues tend to blur, privacy is a social concept, and fraud is a more granular component of privacy. Cryptocurrency is an emerging technology that utilizes encryption methods to create currency units and transfer them outside the realm of the banking system. It is a relatively new technology and therefore has some pending questions. There are still negotiations as to how the currency should be categorized: foreign, domestic, private, commodity, software program, or as an electronic document (Pai, 2015). Cryptocurrency is going to prove useful for organizations in e-commerce. With multiple transactions and payment mediums, cryptocurrency can be an easy method of payment when dealing with different currencies, laws, regulatory bodies, and companies.

Bitcoins, an example of cryptocurrency, is gaining attention in e-markets. Just as PayPal has gained utility, Bitcoin is in the early stages. Bitcoins can be used for a variety of purchases and more companies are accepting them as a form of currency ("Cryptocurrency Trader Launches Super Deal for Bitcoin Sellers", 2015). Signing up for Bitcoin requires entering PayPal or bank information. One must think, if someone is linking their bank account to PayPal, which is linked to Bitcoin, which is then used in many companies and potentially many countries, there are a lot of potential threats to one's financial information. Organizations need to implement the necessary safe guards if they are going to use this technology safely.

CONCLUSION

Technology seems to operate in a separate universe that doesn't have to abide by the law. Technology companies are adamant that they are not legally responsible for the harm their services can cause or the activities of their users ("Eroding Exceptionalism", 2017). Having to monitor their users would be difficult and costly to these companies. Law makers from all parts of the world are considering having to intervene. The technology companies would much rather prefer self-regulation. Urs Gasser, a director and professor at Harvard University, believes that companies indeed have all the information they need to identify bad acting users.

An increase in transparency needs to occur in regards to what monitoring is occurring while consumers conduct their e-transactions. Also, more governmental control of user agreements and online laws in general is necessary. The existing institution of government already provides a stable environment for e-commerce to grow with legal and consumer considerations (Kamel & Hussein, 2001). An additional concern is the speed at which technology evolves compared to the slow reaction of the judicial system (Lawrence, Culjak, & Lawrence, 2003).

Book 4: The World of Business

16

Business Leadership: Methods

Business theories are meaningless if they are not applicable to the real world. There are many different schools of thought in the business field. Leadership is the most important factor for project success (Wu et al, 2012). Leadership has different meanings for different people (Latham, 2014). Pamfilie & Draghici (2012) said that leadership is "the use of influence to encourage participation in achieving set goals" (p. 188). Brown, Brown, & Yocum (2012) offer a functional definition of leadership: "a relationship of influence in which the leader seeks to influence the behavior, attitudes, vision, values or beliefs of another" (p. 896). Part of exhibiting leadership is having a strong desire to improve, being open to new ideas, and listening to feedback (Granko et al, 2013). When studied, it was determined that one leadership approach does not give the best results (Galli & Handley, 2014). There are many approaches to effective leadership, but one approach will not yield the optimal results.

As mentioned before, there are many leadership theories. Some theories even conflict. As opposed to Clark et al (2012) who think that vision and mission statements should be avoided, Bolte (2014) believes that mission statements need to be built strongly and heavily adhered to. Bolte subscribes to the Six Sigma management school of thought. She discusses ten useful tips to implement Six Sigma practices. Her major piece of advice is: initial implementation is met with the most resistance, include everyone's expertise, start with the small and short projects first, and have a backup plan (Bolte, 2014). A high degree of planning and coordination is exhibited by good leaders. Six sigma leadership is one leadership theory that may be employed in teams. Galli and Handley (2014) described shared leadership in teams as leadership that is created when individual members influence other members. The authors also make the point that leaders can usually make any changes they want, but in the end, it matters how the changes are perceived and followed by the employees. Everyone on a team should be able to lead and represent their own point of view.

EMOTIONAL LEADERSHIP
The "Emotional Intelligence of Leaders", a piece by Daniel Goleman, explores the association between emotional intelligence and a leader's ability to effectively manage their organization. Goleman acknowledges that both intelligence and credentials are essential to business management and

leadership, but one cannot overlook the importance of empathy and emotions. These latter aspects are needed because bosses need to interact with their workers to effectively manage a business. The author states that only one-third of the skills needed for leadership are intellectual. Most of the skills needed for effective management are not based in factual knowledge, but rather emotions used to interact with people.

Goleman goes on to explain the biological basis for the brain to reason and express emotions. He discusses how the limbic system and amygdala balance self-control and impulses. Goleman argues that the basis of emotional intelligence relies upon the balance between the thinking brain and the emotional brain. He believes that there are five dimensions of emotional intelligence that are essential for optimal leadership. The dimensions are: self-confidence, self-control, motivating others, showing empathy, and staying connected. Self-control and effective management of emotions are needed to effectively communicate and gain a positive reputation with employees. Managing impulsivity, anger, anxiety, and stress are vital leadership skills.

Self-confidence and self-awareness are critical for self-assessment. Self-assessment is important for improving the state of the organization. Self-control and effective management of emotions are needed to effectively communicate and gain a positive relationship with employees. Employees look to their leader for guidance;

therefore, leaders need to be optimistic and motivating. Along with managing their own emotions, leaders need to understand the emotions of their workers. Empathy shows that the leader cares and creates respect between the worker and the manager. Staying connected and being enthusiastic in the workplace is important. Leaders have much power, including the power to change people's emotions positively or negatively, which directly impacts productivity and the overall morale of the company. At an early age, emotional intelligence develops in children; however, anyone can achieve emotional intelligence by putting in lots of continual effort, implementing organizational support, and understanding how the emotional brain works.

THOUGHT LEADERSHIP

Goleman states that there are three kinds of performance-based classifications in a team setting: poorly performing, well performing, and superlative teams. The poorly performing team is limited by its individual average. The well performing team performs above average. But a superlative team performs better than the best member of the team. Superlative teams work synergistically. This kind of team has been described as "organized genius." Factors that contribute to this kind of team are harmony, trust, and team identification. Being a superlative team is beneficial to a company and should be a goal the company strives for.

Mitch McCrimmon's article, "Thought leadership: a radical departure from traditional, positional leadership", compares aspects of positional leadership and thought leadership. The article maintains that thought leadership is the best way to run a business. The author explains other models of leadership and tries to show that thought leadership is the most effective. Thought leadership is the best model to adopt in businesses where innovation is the key to success. This form of leadership does not rely on managerial elements but rather utilizes knowledge as the driving force. In this model, leadership is neither shared nor distributed. Leadership is held by all members of the organization. The purpose of thought leadership is to challenge the current state of the business (policies, procedures etc.) and to strive for implementing change.

Since there are no managerial elements in thought leadership; there are also no hierarchies. In this model, technical excellence and a member's expertise are valued more than group domination. The rationale of the idea is more important than the implementation of that idea. Once an idea is accepted, it usually leaves the department and goes to another department for the actual implementation. Thought leadership is only successful if people accept the idea. This form of leadership has no boundaries. The idea can originate from a third party outside the organization such as global groups, leadership experts, or relatives of workers. McCrimmon states that thought leadership strives to convince, not to order. Again, this form of leadership is especially important for businesses that need innovation in order to succeed.

CONCLUSION

Research on emotions in business is increasing. Researchers are calling for more research in this area of study (Rafaeli, 2013). One can see that a workplace is always filled with many kinds of emotions. Tähtinen argues that all of the basic emotions, excluding love, are involved in businesses (Tähtinen, 2011). These emotions affect business relationships, professionalism, and can lead to distractions at work. If the basic emotions: joy, surprise, anger, sadness, and fear can be managed, so can the workers. The manager is someone everyone in an organization looks to. The manager has a critical role in the management of these emotions.

Thought leadership is specific to businesses that thrive on innovation. Emotional leadership is applicable across an array of business models. Through working in high stress areas, I feel that emotional leadership is more applicable to businesses. People are emotional beings. If one wants to manage and persuade people, it's logical then, to use an emotional approach. Most businesses do not rely heavily on innovation. Humans are in all businesses and all humans have emotions; therefore, emotional leadership is more useful and effective. Emotions can be a powerful, persuasive tool. A manager is essentially persuading people to do different tasks. If someone is persuaded that the task is necessary to the work flow, they will do it without complaints. This leads to higher productivity. This in the end is not the goal, but it's a step towards the final goal, which is in itself, progress. Since there are no managerial elements in thought leadership; there are also no hierarchies. In this model, technical excellence and a member's expertise are valued more than group domination; therefore humility is an absolute necessity (Francke, 1955). Rationale and analysis of the idea is more important than the actual implementation of that idea. Thought leadership is only successful if people accept the idea.

17

"What we have done for ourselves alone dies with us; what we have done for others and the world remains and is immortal."

- ALBERT PIKE

JACK WELCH OF GENERAL ELECTRIC AND LEADING A NEW ERA

Difficulty of Welch's Challenge

When Jack Welch became Reginald Jones' replacement as CEO at General Electric (GE), Welch was stepping into the shoes of a legend. Jones drove lots of effective change and greatly improved GE overall. Welch had the challenge of perpetuating the change that existed, along with further improving multiple aspects of the organization. Another layer of difficulty that Welch faced is that GE is such a broad company. They have products in numerous industries (ie: lighting, appliances, engines, medical equipment, locomotives) and the connecting markets are usually located in Japan. Even though Jones was a tough act to follow, Welch proved that he was up to the task by successfully implementing effective initiatives and cultural changes.

Initiative Objectives: Late 80s to Early 90s

"Work-Out" and "Best Practices" were two of the major initiatives that Welch launched. His goal for these initiatives was that they would potentiate the desired change in both organizational culture and management. He wanted to create the culture of a small company so that all employees felt that they had a voice. Welch saw the value in GE's service-based segments and in turn focused intangible assets in those areas to grow the already successful sectors that contributed to about 60% of GE's overall revenue. The initiatives proved successful in increasing value, increasing innovation, and improving the organization's overall culture and attitudes.

Six Sigma

Welch implemented most of these initiatives by following Six Sigma methodology. Six Sigma aims to remove defects and improve efficiencies, while utilizing data in order to enhance overall operations. In order to utilize the knowledge of other companies in the industry, GE sought out smart, innovative companies to acquire or merge with. In 1997, GE made 20 acquisitions and joint ventures with other service-related organizations. Due to GE's large investment of $17.5 billion, the company experienced a huge increase in foreign sales. Welch was extremely successful in implementing many new initiatives while engaging the knowledge and assets of other industry leaders.

Defying Pressures of Critics and Remaining Profitable

Modern business practices suggest that GE should separate all of its product lines into many small businesses. Welch refused to do so. Even while hospitalized, he remained adamant that he did not want GE's diverse portfolio broken up. In the end, GE was successful partly due to Welch's defiance of the status quo. Welch's initiatives added great value to the organization. Welch has lead lots of great changes in numerous sectors; however, the quantity may have lessened the quality. Welch led a summit where he heard 108 proposals from GE's employees. He was given very limited time to hear the proposals and deliver a verdict. Welch accepted 100 of the 108 proposals. All of these proposals lead to company-wide initiatives. This was incredibly expensive. It's a lot to be implemented at one time, especially when the organization is already undergoing a severe cultural change. The verdict is still out on the success of these initiatives, but the sheer number has some critics skeptical.

Staffing and Human Resource Concerns

With Welch's large reduction in staff (a 50% decrease) and then subsequently hiring more staff (ie: the new implementation team), the potential for information loss was great which can hinder the future of GE's sustainable operations. Welch hoped to identify employees that did not share the company's vision by using a 5 point rating system that categorized workers according to 4 types of leaders. The fourth type of leader (which delivers on commitments, makes all numbers, but doesn't share company values) Welch would coach. If he could not change their attitude, he would let them go. Furthermore, he only kept staff that he thought directly contributed to the overall value of the company.

This staffing reorganization is rather concerning. Welch, on one hand labels people according to their thoughts on the company's values, while on the other hand, states he wants to rid labels as they hinder organizational culture (ie: hourly employees, salaried employees, etc.). He hand-selected people to fire and drastically purged the company of workers. A major concern of the staffing reduction is that there are less levels of command, giving Welch much more power. He also purged the executive board by creating a "varsity team" of elite stakeholders. He seems to have way too much power and there is a severe lack of checks and balances that limit his power. Lastly, Welch believed that managers should have between 10 and 15 direct reports, contradictory to modern management theory (between 6 and 7 direct reports). This is a disaster waiting to happen. If managers have too many direct reports, there is less control and employees can perform poorly.

Globalization

Upon Welch de-staffing, re-staffing, and then bringing in consultants, in order to meet the company's need for exceptional talent, he pushed GE to move to Phase 3 of their globalization plan. Instead of focusing on global markets, Welch believed the focus should be on expanding efforts to globalize the company's intellect. At the same time, Welch wanted management to focus on improving the company's existing employees. He urged managers to reward and promote the most productive employees. Lastly, Welch wanted each business segment to create its own global strategy. This makes sense since GE's business portfolio is extremely diverse; however, there should be an overall, unifying plan that bridges the gaps between the segments and provides an overall picture of GE's intentions in global markets.

Investment in Employees

Along the lines of rewarding employees appropriately, Welch invested lots of time and money ($45 million) into the renovation of a company plant in Crotonville, NY. He converted it from a management development facility into a place that supports the change and transformational initiatives that Welch was implementing. Welch wanted the employees' report cards to reflect the open, free, and creative environment that is GE. This further supports the boundryless organization that Welch aspired to. He thought that by rewarding employees in their pocketbooks, they would feel a sense of pride and accomplishment.

In addition to rewarding employees more, Welch spent at least 70% of his time dealing with employee issues and developing employees. It is good that Welch wanted to reward employees where rewards are due; however, a CEO is neither a trainer nor a developer. He should have been doing more important things and delegating those initiatives to managers under him. Lastly, Welch should not have been focusing on *what* people got done but rather *how* things got done. Looking at the "how" would have allowed him to identify loopholes in efficiencies and identify opportunities for improvement.

Entering a New Era of GE: Replacing Welch

Welch greatly contributed to the success of GE while he was the CEO. He conquered numerous initiatives that improved upon his predecessor's initiatives. He juggled the mass exodus of staff, the large number of business units, and at the same time approved proposals while managing his subordinates. Welch's successor needs to continue Welch's efforts and follow through with the initiatives that have been implemented.

Welch implemented a strong e-commerce initiative on his way out the door. He communicated that the building

of strong brands, top-ranked product reliability, great ful-
fillment capability, and excellent quality service are key
assets that are needed for e-commerce to be successful.
Ecommerce is on the shoulders of Welch's successor to
see if it has remained successful and sustainable. The major key to the success of Welch's replacement is that he or
she sees the company for what it truly is: a conglomerate
of about 350 business segments.

SATYA NADELLA OF MICROSOFT AND DIVERSITY IN THE WORKPLACE

Microsoft changed CEOs in 2014. There are numerous publications in academic journals and newspapers that show
both skepticism and praise for the new CEO of Microsoft:
Satya Nadella. Microsoft's website contains numerous an-
nouncements and emails from Nadella to his employees
announcing his new visions for the company. Nadella writes
how the technology industry does not care for tradition and
the successful companies must innovate. Their revamped
mission and vision statement, as posted on their website,
boasts of the company enabling people around the globe
to realize their full potential. They want to change the world
by improving access to technology. Microsoft is improving
accessibility to technology by making their devices more
user-friendly for physically disabled users.

Since Nadella became Microsoft CEO in 2014, he has
lead the company away from its failing mobile strategy towards other opportunities such as cloud computing and

Artificial Intelligence (AI) ("Satya Nadella", 2017). Nadella appointed Harry Shum to be in charge of the new AI unit ("What Satya Nadella did at Microsoft", 2017). Although Microsoft is now committing itself to the potential of AI, Google and Amazon started much earlier. With the purchase of LinkedIn in 2016, Microsoft's stock has never been higher ("Satya Nadella", 2017). Nadella says that "technologies come and go, we need a culture that allows you to constantly renew yourself" ("What Satya Nadella did at Microsoft", 2017).

Contrary to some critics, Nadella is a great communicator. In multiple correspondences, Nadella voices excitement and passion that he is a part of a great organization with excellent leaders who are talented and innovative. He believes that diversity is a key aspect of talent and innovation which is critical for the company's success. The company publishes their annual reports, but they are mostly monetary figures that do not correspond to diversity. However, there are figures on the company website that show the demographics of Microsoft's employees. The company has great programs that promote diversity and create a strong community across cultural boundaries. Due to the sheer number of documents that corroborate Microsoft's message, I believe that Microsoft's commitment to diversity and multiculturalism is genuine.

Employee Diversity

On February 4th, 2014 Satya Nadella wrote an email to his employees stating his excitement and beliefs regarding the direction of the company ("Satya Nadella email to employees", 2016). On the Facts About Microsoft page, the company reports their employee's demographics: 71% male, 29% female and the top three ethnicities are approximately reported as: 61% Caucasian, 29% Asian, and 5.1% Hispanic/Latino.

Microsoft promotes inclusion and togetherness on their Global Diversity and Inclusion Homepage. They have Employee Relation Groups (ERGs) for every demographic and group of employee: Asians, Blacks, Disabled, Women, Parents, Hispanic/Latino, and LGBT. Microsoft strives to coordinate programs to promote diversity. Events such as the Asian Leadership and Development Conference (ALDC) and Black History Month are some of the things that ERGs participate in. In addition to the demographic groups for employees, the company reports that they have programs to further the study of computer science at multiple universities for minority students. Microsoft also has a program specifically for encouraging girls to pursue computer science: DigiGirlz. To this day, Microsoft continues to be dedicated to service a diverse population and providing opportunities that they wouldn't have otherwise.

Paying It Forward

Microsoft's former CEO, Bill Gates, has a shared passion with his wife to increase distribution of shared resources all around the world. Bill and Melissa are strong believers that data analytics can help in their international endeavors: "What we don't measure, we don't work on. We haven't measured women" (Murphy, 2017). There is a general, in-advertent bias towards women in lots of surveys. In order to know where to act, provide resources, and gain funding, there must be an understanding of the current situation. That's where data analytics comes in. Without good data, it's hard to get government support. If one can put numbers and statistics in their sentences, it's easier to illustrate the need and know where to dedicate resources.

Use of Microsoft's Products

One of Microsoft's products is Kinect. It is a motion sensor for their gaming counsel Xbox One. There was an academic study done by a collaboration of two science universities in China. It found that the Kinect can be used as a clinical assessment tool to determine a patient's body sway, which can be used to diagnose various diseases (Yueng, Cheng, Fong, Lee, & Tong, 2014). Two other journal articles talked about their institution's utilization of Microsoft SharePoint. One university, the University of Maryland - University College, used the program for cloud computing and the development of an Intranet. Another paper examined how the Manhattan Community College used SharePoint to digitally catalog their data (Eng & Stadler, 2014; Diffin, Chirombo, & Nangle, 2010). Lastly, Taiwanese researchers observed that the utilization of Microsoft Live@Edu Cloud Platform greatly improved Chinese Reading Literacy in junior high school students (Ru-Chu, Chia-Liang, Chih-Cheng, & Shi-Jer, 2013). These are just a few examples of how Microsoft's business is creating an impact on our world.

Conclusion

Microsoft is referenced numerous times in business journals due to its philanthropic work. Microsoft has an Alumni Foundation. It is comprised of former employees of Microsoft. They hold annual engagements to support the Microsoft foundation which funds many programs to encourage people to get into technology careers. The foundation also supports charitable causes to help people with diseases such as HIV, malaria, pneumonia, and tuberculosis. Microsoft's founder Bill Gates is still heavily involved with the foundation. Bill and his wife, in addition to having an interest in increasing healthcare access, also have a passion of getting girls and women interested in technology jobs. Long after Gates' departure as CEO of Microsoft, the company continues its efforts of increasing diversity and expanding access to healthcare.

GINNI ROMETTY OF IBM AND SHIFTS IN TECHNOLOGY

International Business Machines (IBM), also known as "Big Blue", is a technology company that has been around for a long time and has survived numerous changes in technological trends and advancements. The current CEO, Ginni Rometty, was in the spotlight at the turn of the first quarter of the 21st century. As the first woman CEO of IBM, she is in charge of leading IBM through another technological transition in moving towards an age of artificial intelligence, cognitive systems, data analytics, and cloud computing ("Ginni Rometty", 2017). During this time, IBM was selling business segments that generated billions in sales, but they lost money or broke even. Rometty was generating huge earnings in cognitive computing because of the potential of Watson's platform and it's capability to analyze data from hospitals, universities, and businesses. It is obvious why Forbes listed Rometty as the 61st most powerful person in 2016 and the 11th most powerful woman in 2016 ("Ginni Rometty", 2017).

The IBM Legacy

As a technology company, IBM has survived change multiple times over the years. In the mid-1980s, IBM was inventing complex banking systems, office systems, and ATMs (Chafkin, 2016a). In the early 1990s, IBM was forced to reinvent itself if it was to stay relevant. If it didn't, it would've dissolved with all of the other irrelevant technology companies of the time. This is the reason IBM has been thriving for 105 years: the company transforms with the latest technology trends of the time. Ironically, as much as the company has transformed, they still utilize mainframes, an ancient IT infrastructure, in 10% of their business. Mainframes at IBM still run airline systems and currency exchanges. Although IBM has changed over the years, IBM's core values and mission have withstood the test of time.

IBM still resides at the intersection of inventing and applying new technology. Usually technological transitions involve one technology morphing into a more innovative technology of the same type, with the same use, and intention. What's unique about the transition most technology companies are undergoing in the 21st century is that multiple technologies with differing applications spanning numerous industries are simultaneously changing together (Chafkin, 2016a). Big data, cloud computing, mobility, and artificial intelligence are all undergoing innovation at the same time. This has advantageously accelerated change for IBM and its customers.

IBM and Diversity

At the time of all this technological change, there were so many political and social issues that plagued society. Opinions on political parties, women's rights, and gender rights were a point of high contention. During the 2017 Inauguration of the President of the United States, companies voiced their political opinions. This caused people to question their company's commitment to diversity. Rometty restated its commitment to the diversity of its employees. IBM has had a long history of its commitment to diversity. Rometty claims IBM had the idea of equal opportunity eleven years before the Civil Rights Act was passed (Chafkin, 2016a). She also boasts of the company's service of shipping traveling female employees' breast milk who recently had children back to their homes. The CEO restates the company's commitment to keeping women in the workforce. Lastly, on the topic of gender rights, IBM spoke out against North Carolina's bathroom bill. The bill sought to prevent transgender people from using the public bathroom of their choosing. IBM has long been dedicated to LGBT rights. IBM commits to keeping their workplace open to everyone, regardless of their beliefs.

Employee and Company Competition

With the large number of technology companies, certain organizations can find it difficult to cultivate a skilled employee pool. Startups like Google and Facebook are attractive places for people to work. Millennials straight out of college tend to be attracted to these kinds of startups because in mainstream technology, they appear to be on the edge of the "latest-and-greatest" trend. IBM has been around for 105 years and their products do not appear to be in the public spotlight as their technology is typically housed inside another company's product. Rometty views IBM as a "grown-up company" (Walters, 2016). IBM's clients trust the company with their most valuable data and processes (Chafkin, 2016a).

Ginni Rometty says that workers come from Google and Facebook to IBM because they want to make a serious impact on technological advances. The 1.5 million employment applications that IBM receives a year speak to that desire of working for IBM. IBM helps move planes around, uses cognitive systems to create human-computer partnerships, and is working on helping doctors detect cancer. Google works on applications. IBM's CEO Ginni Rometty believes the company is in a great spot to compete in the technology marketplace and its job market.

Artificial Intelligence and Cognitive Systems

The capabilities of IBM's cognitive system platform, Watson, is endless. IBM is working on developing it as a service that it can sell. It runs on an Application Programming Interface (API) housed in the IBM Public Cloud where users can manipulate the code via system tools (Chafkin, 2016a). Artificial intelligence is just one of the fifty things that Watson can do. Machine learning, text-to-speech, speech-to-text, and different analytical engines are just some of Watson's abilities. IBM does not make consumer devices, but rather creates Watson's capabilities to be housed in a device made by another technology company.

One example of IBM creating capabilities is working with Medtronic to create a product that predicts hypoglycemic events in patients three hours in advance of the actual event (Chafkin, 2016a). Another healthcare application is in helping doctors detect cancer in patients that reside in rural areas where few doctors are accessible. Watson Oncology is being deployed in India where there are only 1,000 oncologists per billion people. This is delivering hope to patients that wouldn't normally have access to cancer care. Great advances have been made in oncology. This has led to the increase in number of treatment options for patients. Watson can help mediate doctor's ability to choose the best treatment for the patient the first time. CEO Ginni Rometty doesn't care if people know that Watson is inside these devices. She's confident that IBM's cognitive platform will be able to compete with Apple's Siri and Amazon's Alexa (Walters, 2016). IBM is paving the way with Watson and its applications on personal assistants, healthcare, and everyday life.

Robot Takeover

In the technology circuit, there have been debates and concerning discussions on the implications of robots, or artificial intelligence, gaining abilities and power. Concerns of ethics, privacy, and job availability have stemmed from the increasing abilities of these technologies. IBM CEO Ginni Rometty is convinced that Watson and other cognitive computing platforms will not lead to a robot takeover (Zillman, 2017). Watson has been fed textbooks and medical journals, and then subsequently trained on cancer causes. It can now spot cancers, in some instances, better than human experts.

Rometty believes that Artificial intelligence has the ability to solve some of the "world's most unsolvable problems" (Zillman, 2017). Robots support the human ability, they don't replace it. There are jobs that can currently be replaced with automation, but they're not. Even if the potential exists to replace human jobs with robots, it probably will not occur. Humans play a vital role in building AI's abilities to complete even more complex tasks. Rometty has outlined the company's principles for the cognitive era: purpose, transparency and skills (Zillman, 2017). Companies that possess powerful technologies need to introduce them into society in a responsible way.

New Collar Jobs and Future Aspirations amidst Uncertainty

During the 2017 transition of political power in America, there were many unanswered questions surrounding the future climate of technology, businesses, and jobs. IBM, a company that has been around for 105 years, has seen many periods of change and uncertainty. Education, IT infrastructure, and healthcare are important passions of IBM. There is no other company that is positioned better to offer recommendations on the future of the technology industry. More and more incoming students, parents, and employers are realizing that a college education is not always needed, especially in technology jobs. Not everyone out of high school is emotionally and physically ready to go to a four year college. Even if they are, they often don't know what degree program they want to pursue. IBM's CEO believes a new kind of job is forming: "new collar" jobs. These jobs comprise of expertise in areas such as cybersecurity, data science, artificial intelligence, and cognitive business (Rometty, 2016). The college degree is becoming less of a necessity because vocational training can give prospective employees the needed skills to fill these jobs. Around one-third of people employed at IBM have less than a four-year degree. Rometty is championing for six year public high schools that include traditional high school and community college along with real-world job experience.

As "new collar" jobs expand, the IT infrastructure that supports these operations needs to expand too. These types of jobs involve the processing of massive amounts of data. This can require lots of memory and other storage capacities. The IT infrastructure in America needs to grow to support this. Investments in the Internet of Things (IoT) and Artificial Intelligence (AI) can improve performance. As infrastructure gets bigger and smarter, the need for cybersecurity also increases. IBM wants America to build big IT infrastructure in a smart, methodical manner.

Healthcare

IBM has demonstrated their commitment to improving healthcare through their cognitive computing platform: Watson. In India, Watson Oncology has drastically improved healthcare delivery even in its early phases. IBM is one of the largest employer-sponsored health plans in the United States. The company has 15 specific ideas on how America can change the healthcare system to save more than $900 billion over ten years and an additional trillion dollars solely due to fraud prevention (Rometty, 2016). Some of these ideas include using data analytics to reduce fraudulent Medicare claims, improving the exchange of health records among providers, and leveraging the government's purchasing power to lower the cost of drugs and healthcare.

American Veterans are struggling to get quality healthcare. Many citizens are upset that military men and women go overseas to fight for their country, only to return home and not be able to receive decent healthcare for injuries, mental and physical, that occurred during battle. More must be done to ensure American veterans get the best medical care possible. IBM started a pilot program in conjunction with the Department of Veterans Affairs (VA) to help oncologists treat thousands of veterans via precise medical treatment and genomic analysis (Rometty, 2016). This technology and delivery of care is powered by IBM's Watson.

Conclusion

IBM has around 150 offices around the world that are open workspaces that promote small team collaboration (Chafkin, 2016a). IBM is the world's largest commercial research organization in the world. They own 12 labs around the globe that employ more than 3,000 researchers that comprise 10% of all the Mathematic PhD scholars in the world. There is no other company that is more equipped to take on a new form of computing that utilizes massive amounts of data. IBM has the power and resources to transform the industry (Walters, 2016; Chafkin, 2016a). From being an IBM engineer in the early 80s, to working her way up to CEO in 2012, Ginni Rometty will not be having her tenure defined as being the woman CEO of IBM, but rather as being the leader of cognitive, transformative computing.

TIM COOK OF APPLE AND BUSINESS ACTIVITIES

Apple is the most profitable business; it obtained over $9 billion in net income the last quarter of 2016 ("Tim Cook", 2017). The fact that Apple is a leader in entertainment, design, and technology positions Apple to be able to lead the industry of startup firms. However, iPhone sales make up 60% of the company's sales when it was at an all-time high. Currently, it is lower. Apple is a growing technology company in the United States that thrives off of innovation. Apple utilizes many business activities such as business intelligence, enterprise resource planning (ERP), customer relationship management (CRM), data mining, and intelligent systems to contribute to the success and longevity of the organization. Effectiveness and productivity are central to all business activities. By turning raw data into useful data that businesses can use, organizations can react to changing markets and thrive in their current environment. Apple uses these business methodologies to track, monitor, and record user activity. Finally, the recorded data is then used to implement changes that will positively benefit the customers and generate revenue for the organization.

Business Intelligence

Business Intelligence (BI) ensures that technology is implemented correctly and yields the most benefit to the organization. Enterprise resource planning (ERP) uses software to integrate information from multiple applications and platforms. Customer relationship management (CRM) is used to interact with potential, current, and future customers in an automated fashion. Data mining is a methodology used to search multiple databases to generate new information that is then used to analyze how the business is operating and how it can be improved. Intelligent systems are machines that have internet-enabled computers connected to them to carry out physical functions. All of these business activities, if implemented correctly, can benefit the organization by providing data-driven decisions. The ultimate goal of the business activities is to utilize the collected data to improve operations.

Business Intelligence (BI) incorporates techniques to turn raw data into meaningful information to benefit the business. As a result, it promotes efficiency and productivity while providing the information that organizations need to achieve their goals. Apple uses BI to track the popularity of songs and artists in iTunes. Other types of data that Apple utilizes include:

- Total number of movies downloaded
- Total amount of revenue generated by movie downloads

- Number of movies downloaded by genre, country, region, state, city, age group, etc.
- Amount of revenue generated by movie downloads across these dimensions
- Number of movies downloaded and amount of revenue generated from sales versus rentals
- Amount paid for the rights to sell or rent each movie
- Download and revenue rates for competitors in the streaming media market (e.g., Amazon, Google, Netflix)
- Overall increases in the number of users purchasing or renting digital movies versus discs

(Yonce, 2015)

No matter what data is looked at, the goal is always the same: to utilize data to create positive and productive actions. BI is most concerned with how technology can aid the organization in becoming more efficient and profitable to meet the goals of the organization.

For example, a goal for iTunes is to optimize revenue from their digital sales and distribution platform. This optimization of revenue is done by documenting who is downloading what on which device. Broadly, Apple tries to make processes more efficient and compares metrics against the goals. Sources of data to get these metrics include: billing data, iTunes content data, supplier data, an independent analysis of competitor data, and an independent analysis of overall market data (Yonce, 2015). Having clearly defined metrics will help limit the number of possible data sources and the size of the resulting data set that must be analyzed.

Enterprise Resource Planning (ERP)

Enterprise resource planning (ERP) is using software to integrate information across multiple applications. In addition, ERP can also be integrated with other methodologies and techniques. Some researchers have been examining the effect of integrating Lean Six Sigma and ERP (Powell, Riezebos, & Strandhagen, 2013). Lean Six Sigma and ERP aim to increase productivity in order to problem solve and improve processes. Lean depends on data to problem solve and continuously improve. Organizations are increasing the integration of their products with multiple platforms (Brodkin, 2009; Eddy, 2009). This increased integration allows for on-the-go access to live dashboards that display ERP, CRM, and ecommerce operational data via Apple iOS. Some features of NetSuite's ERP app are customer fields, customer records, role-based security, and custom dashboard elements. Visibility.net also launched its application on iOS ("Visibility to Bring Full ERP", 2010). Users can now access transactional functions and reports from their own internal systems along with business intelligence features. ERP focuses on continuity across software and platforms.

Customer Relationship Management (CRM)

Customer relationship management (CRM) is using computers to automatically interact with potential, current, and future customers. Apple is using CRM systems to integrate payment platforms. Apple Genius is a payment and program acceptance software that integrates all payment types, mobile wallets, and mobile commerce solutions. Major features of the solution are unlimited choice, unified security, open access, maximum flexibility ("Merchant Warehouse", 2012). Ultimately, the goal is to drive incremental growth and deliver powerful mobile commerce solutions. Due to the increase in usage of CRM, software that manages customer relationships is being developed across all platforms ("Webfortis and Microsoft Announce Apple Watch App", 2015). Apps and computer programs are created so that CRM can be done from anywhere, anytime, on any platform.

Data Mining

Data mining is a technique to examine extensive databases to create new information. Apple's utilization of data mining is increasing. The company applied for a patent for a technology they have developed. The patent describes techniques, methods, systems, and programs for point data mining ("Merchant Warehouse", 2012). The technology is used to determine geographic coordinates of a user's device. The technology utilizes GPS and wireless signal triangulation to ensure that the coordinates the program returns are accurate. Cross checking is done with the user's billing address.

Apple, Privacy, and the FBI

In 2015 at a rented banquet hall in San Bernardino, CA, a married couple killed 14 people and injured 22 in an act of Islamic terrorism. A few hours later, police chased the suspects and engaged in a shootout where both suspects were killed. An iPhone was recovered in their vehicle. The Federal Bureau of Investigation (FBI) opened an investigation. During the course of the investigation, they tried many times to unlock the iPhone but failed. Apple prides themselves on protecting their customer's privacy. However, a federal judge ordered Apple to create a special tool to allow the FBI to break through the security protections on the iPhone (Kiser, 2016). Apple didn't want to create such a thing and said it wasn't even possible. Meanwhile, the US government made it seem like it would be a cheap, easy thing to create. The White House refused to force technology makers to install backdoors. In the end, national security officials found a way to gain access to the most secure consumer devices such as Apple's iPhone. Despite the orders from the US government, Apple did not create a backdoor because they stuck to their commitment to protect their customers' privacy.

The incident lead to a debate about the government's ability to force companies to comply with hacking requests. Some politicians thought that it's a matter of national security and companies need to create a way for them to hack into their own devices. Something as simple as a universal code, that only the company knows, that can allow an infinite number of login attempts rather than locking up and erasing the phone after the attempts. This was such a topic of discussion that it showed up in an episode of *Law and Order: Special Victims Unit*. The storyline of the episode was similar to the San Bernardino incident where a terrorist's burner phone was found and the police could not unlock it. In the episode, the Assistant District Attorney (ADA) explains to the judge that the court needs to compel the manufacturer to unlock the phone so that a terrorist attack can be prevented. The judge notes that it's a highly unusual request and questions the ADA on alternative options. None of which are viable. The data of the terrorist threat is not in the cloud and only exists on the phone. The judge also notes that hundreds of phones are awaiting decryption and are being appealed by the manufacturer. Reluctantly, the judge grants the order.

The manufacturer of the phone doesn't comply with the court order. The ADA cites the All Writs Act of 1789, but the company's lawyer argues the act does not allow the court to force a private company to aid in a criminal investigation. He goes on to explain that the reason for their company's success is that their customers know the company's products are secure. If the company created a piece of software to unlock one phone, it would unlock all of them and cause a threat to customers' security and national security. The company, like Apple, is protecting the security of everyone involved.

Apple's Augmented Reality

Due to Apple's stagnant growth in iPhone sales, the tech company needs to find another product that can help them continue to grow. That's where Augmented Reality (AR), more commonly known as Virtual Reality (VR), comes in. AR is expected to shift how people use electronic devices and therefore could easily cause iPhone sales to plummet even further. In order for Apple to enter into this potential market, they have hired talent from some of the best technology firms, including: Facebook, Microsoft, Dolby, and THX (Gurman, 2017). Apple has also acquired some AR software companies to aid in this endeavor: Metaio, FlyBy Media Inc., and Rockwell. There is absolutely a market in AR. Pokémon Go demonstrated this when it generated $1 billion within the first 6 months after its release (Russell, 2017). Apple is positioned the best to dominate this young market.

Store Competition

Apple's App Store grew 22% over 2016 and reached $24 billion in revenue (Webb, 2017). With the company's leveling off of hardware sales, it can't afford to neglect opportunities in its service division. Apple has a history of rejecting developer's applications and if Apple accepted it they didn't provide data on consumer usage. The CEO believes that their service division will double by 2021. It used to be that developers would wait weeks for decisions from the App Store. With Apple's improvements, they only wait a few days or hours. In addition, Apple now provides better user data to the developer. This is important because Apple's competition provided detailed statistics on consumer's subscriptions and cancellations. Lastly, a seemingly basic feature was added to the App Store: being able to respond to customer reviews (Webb, 2017). Whether it's AR or App Store development, Apple continuously seeks to implement improvements based on market trends and customer feedback.

Conclusion

Every Apple iPhone ad displays the time as 9:41am, the time Steve Jobs unveiled it in 2007 ("Apple Facts", 2015). Because Apple computers implement methodologies from each of the types of business activities, the company has prospered and obtained much success and innovation. In fact, these methodologies and technologies all help Apple to integrate multiple projects, platforms, and software that ultimately use all of the data they have to make smarter business decisions. Apple is going to continue to utilize the tools to continuously improve and capture more sectors of the market. Overall, this leads to increased effectiveness and productivity while allowing for long-term organizational sustainability through innovation.

SUNDAR PICHAI OF GOOGLE AND THE BUILDING OF A MASSIVE STARTUP

Even though Google has expanded way beyond the size of a startup, it continues to ensure that its employees have the capacity to create and innovate like a startup. Project Loon and Google Fiber are two projects that were a result of employee innovation. The projects are unique, their goals are meaningful, and they are beneficial to Google's customer base. Google Fiber is similar to Project Loon but Fiber is more focused on the speed of the internet. These projects can be merged as their premises are the same. In addition, Project Loon is more difficult to sustain in the long term.

Google's unique approach, "Launch and Iterate", seeks to compare its innovation to other technology companies. Almost all of Google's products roll out as beta versions before they are completely released to the public. Google has a few different ideologies when it comes to creating and sustaining innovation. The 70/20/10 innovation model, the "10 things", and innovation time off policies all aid in Google's initiative of sustainable innovation. During Google's extensive 20 interview process, Google recruiters search for the right mixture of skills, agility, and entrepreneurial drive. This methodology of recruiting top talent allows Google to innovate and grow within their industry. Google competes with its competitors by offering better services and acquiring complementary companies via vertical integration.

Even though investors continue to be concerned about Google's high investment in innovating products that may not be successful in the market or even get into the market, Google's stock continues to rise. Google has some work to do to boost the confidence of their investors when it comes to the amount of resources that Google dedicates to innovation. The company has implemented a business model that stresses innovation and technological advances. They gain profits by decreasing costs and engaging in competition with their industry rivals.

Google's Innovation Model

Google's eight pillars of innovation aid Google in maintaining its innovation. In addition to the pillars, Google looks for new ideas for continuous innovation (Purkayastha & Srinivasa Rao, 2014). Even though Google has expanded way beyond the size of a startup, it continues to ensure that its employees have capacity to innovate and create. For Project Loon, the technology may need to be rethought as balloons circling the stratosphere may not be sustainable in the long term and may be a security concern.

One of Google's unique approaches is "Launch and Iterate". It seeks to compare its innovation to other technology companies. Almost all of Google's products are beta versions before they "roll into production". For example, Google Moderator and Tip Jar were created because of feedback from users. This aligns with Google's model of "perfect it before you sell it". Google utilizes lead users to critique its product before Google introduces it to the market.

Entrepreneurial Spirit

Google can keep the entrepreneurial spirit alive by strictly adhering to their "10 things" (Purkayastha & Srinivasa Rao, 2014). The most important ones that contribute to the entrepreneurial spirit are: keep allowing employees to innovate, don't tell employees what they should be innovating, learn from mistakes and failed products, and launch new projects. Setting time aside for innovation can also be crucial in ensuring that Google keeps the spirit alive. The 70/20/10 innovation model is a concise model that's easy to implement. Also, the innovation time off, where employees get 1 day a week to work on innovation, can support Google's innovation efforts.

Cultivation of Talent, Innovation, and Competition

Google has demonstrated its ability to cultivate talented workers. The company's selection process contains 20 extensive interviews. During these interviews, Google recruiters search for the right mixture of skills, agility, and entrepreneurial drive. The recruiting of top talent allows Google to sustain their innovation initiatives and grow in their industry. In addition to the recruitment of talent, Google is great at competing with its competitors. For example, when Google launched Gmail, it offered users 100 times more storage than any other free webmail platform that was offered at the time. Another way that Google competes is through acquisitions. In 2011, Google acquired Motorola for its hardware resources. This allowed Google to compete with companies like Apple who produce both software and hardware.

Business Model

A business model seeks to identify successful operation practices, revenue sources, customers, products, and financing. Johnson, Christensen, and Kagermann state that there are four components to a successful business model: customer value proposition, profit formula, key resources, and key processes (2008). Apple has been successful with their business model that integrates three areas: hardware, software, and service. It seems simple and concise, but not all companies can successfully implement the model. Google has implemented a business model that stresses innovation and technological advances. They gain profits by decreasing costs and competing with their competitors by producing innovative technologies. The innovation succeeds when the product meets a need and customers find value in the product. The cost of innovation and the return on investment of those products are difficult to balance. Some investors think Google is spending too much on innovation.

Google is not the typical company in terms of investments, stakeholders, and stock. They have been a private company until recently. They thrive on creativity and access to free, public information. Contrary to the current structure of public businesses that focus public ownership on historical objectives, Google restructured their firm to protect itself from innovation prevention and differential characteristics ("Letters from the Founders", 2004). Google provides most services for free, while improving the lives of the masses to do things that matter. The goal of Google's release of free services is to bridge the digital divide. AdSense does this by funding a huge variety of on-line advertisements that couldn't otherwise be published. Gmail was released initially with 5 gigabytes (GB) of free storage when the competition only offered 1 GB. This is Google's differentiator.

Google's biggest hurdle in going public is acceptance of its costly innovation. Stakeholders are convinced that Google is wasting money on innovative products that never go to market. Google conducts thousands of working hours on "test products", or experiments that never go to fruition. They have a point as "X", Google's innovation line, lost around $3.6 billion in 2015 (Chafkin & Bergen, 2016). Another project of Google's, Project Loon, seeks to create a fleet of hot air balloons that provide wireless internet to billions of people. Regardless of the innovation, high profit, and extreme potential that Google faces, like Uber, they are having a staffing problem. Top executives from "X" are leaving the company: 2 project leads from Project Loon; an engineer from Project Wing; and the CEOs of Google's telecommunications company, capital venture segment, and the smart thermostat division (Chafkin & Bergen, 2016).

There are some critics that think Google is not able to balance innovation and their core revenue: search advertising. Some go as far as saying that Google is an "advertising company with a bunch of hobbies" (Chafkin & Bergen, np, 2016). Other critics don't hesitate to point out that at periods of Google's history, there were duplicate efforts. At one point, Google had two music subscription services (YouTube Red and Google Play Music), two venture capital groups (GV and CapitalG), two operating systems (Chrome and Android), and two advanced research labs (X and ATAP). At the same time, Google's fiber optic internet business was met with difficulties in permission to dig holes and lay fiber.

Conclusion

Google faces an extremely difficult task of balancing discipline and freedom. The "X" lines of business open Google up to scrutiny from investors. The risk of losing profits to fund possibly profitable products that may not bring in profit is not the typical strategy. Innovation can bring great revenue streams into any business, but when they're losing steam, there are only two options: "being flogged into innovation or taking your hands off the wheel" (Chafkin & Bergen, np, 2016). Part of what makes Google work is its picturesque picnic tables where its developers fly drones and self-driving cars navigate the campus. Typically

Google employees operate under the ordinary standards of Googleplex. "If we're working on a really huge problem," says Teller, "that motivates people to come here, and it motivates them to stay. That's very real. That's not a marketing thing for Google. It's why this place works" (Chafkin & Bergen, np, 2016). Even though investors continue to be concerned about Google's high investment in innovating products that may not be successful in the market, Google's stock continues to rise. There seems to be a disjoint between the amount that Google is spending on innovation and its ranking on lists of most innovative companies. From 2011 to 2013, Google dropped 40 ranks on Forbes' list of *Most Innovative Companies in the World* (Purkayastha & Srinivasa, 2014). Google needs to boost the confidence of their investors by reassuring them that innovation and costs are being appropriately balanced.

TRAVIS KALANICK OF UBER AND CORPORATE DAMAGE CONTROL

Ride sharing companies have shown interest in the Google Car. Other car companies like Ford, Volvo, and Tesla are also interested in the technology (Chafkin, 2016b). The ride sharing service Uber has expressed interest in using driverless cars for their service as it may help them in gaining space in competitive marketplaces such as China. Didi, the Chinese Uber equivalent, is worth $35 billion and is in 400 Chinese cities which accounts for 80% of all taxis in China. The success of a startup in China is dependent on the startup's connection to the Big 3 (Alibaba, Tencent, and Baidu). Didi and Uber fought in the marketplace until Uber left (Alba, 2015). A self-driving car would help Uber differentiate and compete with existing companies in places with high barriers of entry like China.

Detrimental Public Relations and Regulations

Uber encountered a major public relations issue when a former employee went to a blog to disclose Uber's failure to address her sexual harassment complaint. This was compounded when an Uber driver leaked a tape of Uber's CEO, Travis Kalanick, arguing with him over fare cuts. The third and final incident came when sources revealed that Uber secretly uses software to ensure their drivers don't drive city officials that may be trying to spot drivers violating local regulations ("Hard Driving", 2017).

In addition to facing this public scrutiny, Uber is juggling regulation violations. Courts in Europe are trying to determine if Uber is a transport company or a digital service. Uber has been getting by as a digital service so that it doesn't have to comply with strict licensing, insurance, and safety rules. A ruling from a Seattle court allowed Uber drivers to join a union. A British court is deciding if Uber needs to pay a value-added tax ("Hard Driving", 2017). Regulation is proving to be a major hurdle for Uber.

Conclusion

There is a lot of uncertainty in Uber's future. How Uber gets through the court rulings and sexual harassment allegations will determine Uber's future. During this time, if Uber's technical staff seek other employment opportunities, the performance of Uber's application could be at risk. Uber is basing its future livelihood on its development of driverless cars. A company that is competing with these efforts, Waymo, is suing Uber for their lidar technology ("Hard Driving", 2017; Chafkin & Bergen, 2017). It's important that Uber resolves this suit as its future is dependent on it and the first company that goes to market with a driverless car will be able to outcompete Uber by shuttling passengers without paying drivers. In most cases like this, the company getting sued settles for a large sum of money. The lawsuits, risk of staff retention, and regulation dictate Uber's future.

18

Frivolous Lawsuits, High Temperatures, and Burnt Customers

Frivolous lawsuits are clogging the American court system. People are suing companies, of any size, for exaggerated damages they feel that they have incurred. Dramatizations and misinterpreted laws are utilized to win these kinds of cases. Large amounts of money are being asked of companies to compensate for mental suffering, hospital bills, inconvenience, and discomfort. These amounts are completely disproportionate to the cost that the plaintiffs endured.

For instance, a high school student attempted to jump over a volleyball net and broke his neck. He then sued the gym teacher. On one hand, the boy should not have tried to jump over the net, but later it was found that the gym teacher left the room for a long period of time (Enghagen & Gilardi, 2002). The judgment went in favor of the boy due to the negligence of the teacher demonstrated by the teacher leaving the room and abandoning his duties of supervising his students.

Some other cases include an armed mugger who was shot in the back by a police officer as he fled the scene. It was later ruled that police officers cannot shoot fleeing suspects unless the suspect poses a threat to the officer or others. At first glance, these cases may seem frivolous, but upon delving further, these cases hold some legitimacy. Another example of a frivolous lawsuit is when a customer was eating a McDonald's hamburger and as the pickle dropped onto her lap, it hit her chin leaving burns on her chin. The customer sued McDonald's for lost wages, medical bills, and pain and suffering. There have also been multiple cases involving the temperature at which restaurants serve their coffee. These companies include Starbucks, Motor City Bagels, and McDonald's. The rulings have determined that the companies' coffee was "excessively hot" and "unreasonably dangerous" (Enghagen & Gilardi, 2002).

McDonald's has been the center of numerous cases like those previously mentioned. A customer filed a case against McDonald's in regards to the temperature at which they serve their coffee. Liebeck vs. McDonald's will be examined in this paper. Another example of a "frivolous" lawsuit is Pearson vs. Chung. This case involved a dry cleaner that lost a client's pants. Pearson, an administrative judge, represented himself and initially sued for $64 million, which included the fees to represent him. The legitimacy of events leading up to the ruling and the ruling itself will be further examined in this paper.

THE FACTS

In the case of Liebeck vs McDonald's, Liebeck sued McDonald's for damages caused to her by the 49 cent cup of coffee that she ordered. In 1994, Liebeck, an 81 year old grandmother, went through the McDonald's drive-thru in the passenger seat of her Ford Probe. Her grandson was driving. She ordered a cup of coffee. Liebeck's grandson proceeded to pull over and allowed his grandmother to add cream and sugar (Browning, 2011). As she put the coffee cup between her knees, she lifted the lid and the coffee spilled all over her lap. Liebeck was wearing cotton sweatpants which caused prolonged exposure to the scolding beverage resulting in third-degree burns.

Her thighs, butt, and groin got burned. The burns caused her to be hospitalized for eight days and cost her $11,000 (Tennissen, 2007). She initially sued McDonald's for $2.7 million for punitive damages. The trial judge decreased the amount from $2.7 million to $480,000. Both Liebeck and McDonald's appealed this amount. Liebeck felt the judge lowered the initial amount too much and McDonald's thought the amount was still too high. In the end, the case settled for an undisclosed, confidential amount (Browning, 2011).

In the case of Pearson vs Chungs, Pearson, an administrative law judge, took his pants to the Chungs' shop to have the waistline expanded on June 2005 ("Pearson v. Chung", 2005). The cost was to be $10.50 (Sullivan, 2007). The business lost the pants and informed Pearson. After Pearson was not satisfied with the result of going to the Chungs' business, Custom Cleaners, the owners tried to pawn off another pair of pants to Pearson. Mr. Pearson was not happy with the service he received from Custom Cleaners and sued the Chungs.

Pearson initially sued for $64 million. The court later lowered the settlement to $54 million. Finally the court dismissed the case in August 2007 (Sullivan, 2007). As a result of the lawsuit, the Chungs had many expenses. They had to pay these expenses accrued during the lawsuit using donations and family funds.

THE ISSUES

Due to the severity of Liebeck's burns, she was taken to the hospital. She was assessed to have third-degree burns on six percent of her skin and had less-severe burns on over sixteen percent of her skin (Amelinckx, 2011). Liebeck was in the hospital for eight days and had skin grafting done to help heal her burns. Due to her hospital stays, she sued McDonald's for $11,000 in medical bills and $5,000 from not being able to perform her job duties as a department store clerk.

McDonald's claimed that they serve their coffee at high temperatures because that is the way that their customers like it; therefore, they refused to lower the temperature in the future. McDonald's believed that the burns were a result of Liebeck's negligence and therefore they were not liable for the burns. McDonald's refused to settle on multiple attempts because the case lacked merit (Seabury, 2012). In the past ten years there have been 700 people making similar claims about McDonald's coffee being too hot. McDonald's response is that 700 is an insignificant number compared to how many cups of coffee have been sold in that same timeframe (Tennissen, 2007). McDonald's does not see the temperature of their coffee as an issue.

The major motif in Pearson's case is that there were two signs outside of the Custom Cleaners store that read "satisfaction guaranteed" and "same day service." Pearson was not satisfied because he did not receive his pants with the specified alterations that he wanted. He also was offered someone else's pants to compensate for the losing of his by the owners. Pearson believed that because the signs were presented to him, and the statements were not met by the owners, fraud was committed.

APPLICATION OF THE LAW

There is a major lack of laws that specifically apply to these cases. Literature shows that there is no customer consensus on how hot they prefer their coffee to be served; therefore, it is difficult for the plaintiff to comment on the temperature of the coffee as it is a matter of personal preference (Borchgrevink, 1998). It has also been shown that extreme temperatures can cause burns, cellular damage, and death to consumers. The plaintiffs claimed "gross negligence" and that the coffee was "defectively manu-factured", "unreasonably dangerous", and "excessively hot" (Enghagen et al, 2002; Tennissen, 2007). It was estab-lished that coffee should be served no hotter than 140°F (Tennissen, 2007).

Personal-injury cases are regulated by individual states. According to Enghagen & Gilardi (2002), some basic ques-tions remain regardless of the state that has jurisdiction:

1. Was the product defective?
2. Was the product made in an unreasonably danger-ous way?
3. Was the plaintiff aware of the risks associated with the product?
4. Did the defendant have obligations to warn the plaintiff? If so, were the warnings given and were they adequate?
5. Did the product meet applicable industry and gov-ernment safety standards?

These questions are critical in determining the legitimacy of the plaintiff's claim. Applying questions to the Liebeck vs McDonald's are as follows:

1. The product was not defective.
2. The coffee was exceedingly hot and therefore un-reasonably dangerous.

3 and 4. The complainant was made aware of the risks in the form of the "Caution: Hot!" warning label.

5. The coffee was not contaminated and it did not contain another substance other than coffee. Other than that, the industry regulations are vague.

It is possible to make a coffee too hot for human consumption that can cause burns to someone's organs (Borchgrevink, 1998). The plaintiff may not have been aware of the risks. A warning may not have been printed on the cup and if there was one printed, Liebeck may not have seen it. McDonald's is obligated to inform their customers in some way that their coffee is hot and they should be careful. The currently small printed label may not be sufficient warning to the consumer. The product met industry standards. According to the above criteria, McDonald's is not at fault because they served a safe product to the customer.

In Pearson vs Chung, Pearson was not aware of the risks associated with the service he was purchasing. The Chungs did not inform him of the potential for his pants to get misplaced. There was no written agreement stating what should happen if something like this were to happen. The cleaners should be obligated to inform the customer of this scenario. The Chungs are at-fault because they did not deliver their promised services.

Pearson sued Custom Cleaners for $67 million because they lost his pants. This amount was later lowered to $54 million. Even though Pearson represented himself in court, he also sued for $542,000 in legal fees which were included in the amount of $67 million (Goldstein, 2007). The District of Columbia Consumer Protection Act was applied to this case. Mr. Pearson's argument was that the Chung's committed fraud because they did not deliver a service that they stated they would. The lawsuit had merit based on mental suffering, inconvenience, and discomfort caused to Pearson by the Chungs' business.

Pearson claimed the Chungs committed fraud on a historical scale which was executed by the malicious business owners who had no intention of delivering on those services (Sabar & Lee, 2007). The distinction between intention and delivery was important to this case. The Chungs did not intend to lose Mr. Pearson's pants even though Mr. Pearson believes the Chungs had no intention of performing their stated services. This is why the judge dropped the case.

THE DECISION OF THE JUDGE AND JURY

McDonald's put up a fight. They refused many settlements. The case went to trial. The jury was made of six men and six women. They found Liebeck twenty percent at fault so they reduced the settlement accordingly. The settlement was $640,000 plus $2.7 million in punitive damages. McDonald's filed an appeal for this decision. Three months later, in late November, both parties settled for a confidential amount before the appeal was decided. The conclusion of the case was that coffee served at McDonald's is more likely to cause serious injury than coffee served from any other establishment (Tennissen, 2007). Therefore, McDonald's was partly at-fault.

In the Pearson case, the defense presented Mr. Pearson as a man of financial hardships and recent divorce. The defense claimed that Pearson still had a grudge against the Chungs' over another pair of lost pants in 2002. The defense did not stop there; they also claimed that Pearson was using his knowledge of the DC legal justice system to exploit non-English-speaking immigrants who worked more than seventy hours per week to live the American dream (Sabar & Lee, 2007). There has also been a correlation between high award settlements causing the jury to be conservative on the future rulings of cases. The fact that a judge allows such a case in a trial court taints the jury to think that the case has some merit even if it may not (Seabury, 2012).

In the end, the case went to trial and a superior court judge ruled in favor of the Chungs. Pearson filed an appeal. The Chungs incurred more than $100,000 in legal fees which were paid by fundraisers and donations (Sabar & Lee, 2007). Due to the loss of customers, the Chungs had to close two out of their three dry cleaning stores.

The Ruling

The predominant law that was applied to these cases was the District of Colombia Consumer Protection Act. This act is long and ambiguous; it does not include a "catchall prohibition of unfair or deceptive practices" (Yohay, 1977, p.644-645). The draftsman of the act knew that specific provisions would be a challenge for the agency to write, but it would give more direction to people trying to enforce it. General, nonspecific provisions would be easier to write but would be subjected to much variation in interpretation. That is the current state of the act: ambiguity (Yohay, 1997). This can be good or bad depending on the case and the two conflicting perspectives.

Due to this ambiguity, the law is difficult to use in practice. For the McDonald's case, the judge made a good decision. Liebeck suffered burns and time off of work due to the way the company presented their product. Because of this, Liebeck should have been awarded money. However, the amount of money was quite large. There is no proof that Liebeck incurred that amount of injury to warrant that high of a settlement. The point of a settlement is to get the victim back to the state that they were in prior to the incident. A small fraction of Liebeck's settlement could do just that. The judge applied the law correctly, but the amount was not proportional to the nominal damages that the plaintiff suffered.

In Pearson vs Chungs, the case was dismissed. Mr. Pearson had a good argument regarding fraud and the signs that hung outside of Custom Cleaners. The signs stated that the company would provide a service in a way that satisfies the customer. The Chungs did not do that. If someone claims fraud was committed, they also need to prove intent. The Chungs did not intend to lose the pants and cause Mr. Pearson harm; therefore, the judge was correct in dismissing the case as misplacing clothing is usually not intentional and can happen to anyone.

Ethics

The ethical and legal issues overlap in these two cases. Ethical issues are ones that only deal with what one should or should not do. They are solely based on a social, unspoken norm. Legal issues are ones that align with or contradict the law. Ethical and legal issues may overlap or conflict with each other. Sometimes an action may be ethical but not legal. It is the moral responsibility of the plaintiffs to not make false accusations. All parties, legally and morally, need to tell the truth under oath. Neither tampering nor falsifying evidence is good practice in the court of law. Liebeck and Pearson should only claim the monetary damages that they have incurred from the incident. The lawyers need to present accurate evidence and persuade the jury of the correct side of the case, not just their client's side. All parties have the moral responsibility of being ethical and behaving in a manner that allows the right verdict to be reached.

FRIVOL-OSITY

Both of these cases, at first glance, may seem frivolous. Upon looking further into the cases, there is some legal merit to the arguments. Custom Cleaners and McDonald's have had multiple cases filed against them due to similar events. The case could have been easily prevented. McDonald's could have learned from previous cases against them, and the Chungs could have found a better organization scheme. Because of this, the plaintiffs have legal merit in their arguments as these cases were absolutely preventable.

However, the amount of money that the plaintiffs are suing for in these cases are what makes them frivolous. There are very few laws that specifically apply to these cases, and none of them specify amounts that victims are entitled to. Victims should be compensated for their pain and suffering and hospital bills. The frivolous part is when plaintiffs sue for millions of dollars and their lost wages and hospital bills amount to $15,000 at the most. The amount that the plaintiffs sue for and are awarded should be proportional to the damages caused by the defendant.

PREVENTION AND ADVICE

The McDonald's case could have been avoided by not making the coffee so hot. There have been previous cases similar to this filed against McDonald's. This case is the biggest settlement so far. McDonald's has made sure to have cups that warn the customer that the contents are hot. Not all customers read the writing on the cup. Therefore, the only way to truly prevent this from happing in the future is to lower the temperature of the coffee. This can be done by modifying the coffee maker or having a set amount of time that the coffee must sit after being brewed, so that it cools down to a less harmful temperature.

The dry cleaner case is a little more difficult to prevent. The operations at Custom Cleaners are unknown; therefore, it is hard to say where a break in the system occurred that allowed the owners to lose a piece of Mr. Pearson's clothing. Maybe the shop is too small which caused clothes to be stacked on top of each other and lost easily. Also, labeling the clothes with the customer's names could allow for better record keeping. Lastly, the system in which the store operates could have caused the error. It is possible that the Chungs need to change the way in which they do business. Better organization of the shop, labeling of clothing, and procedures could prevent this case from happening in the future.

CONCLUSION

Regardless of the fact that Liebeck won against the McDonald's corporation, other plaintiffs in similar coffee cases have lost. These include defendants that could prove that liquid burns requiring medical attention are not the responsibility of the company (Enghagen & Gilardi, 2002). The previously mentioned questions by Enghagen & Gilardi are difficult to answer in these types of cases. Topics of obligation, standards, and rights are important to these cases. It is the responsibility of the plaintiff to prove not only that the defendant had an obligation to either inform or provide services in a certain way, but also that they did not meet that obligation.

Some other examples of seemingly "frivolous" cases are when a customer renting a room from a hotel sued the owners of the hotel because the hot temperature of the shower caused the plaintiff to fall in the tub. The hotel claimed that it was the responsibility of the plaintiff to inform the hotel of this issue at checkout which the plaintiff did not. The jury ruled that the hotel owed $15,000 to the customer, but the judge reduced the settlement to $9,000 (Enghagen & Gilardi, 2002).

Starbucks has also been involved in cases regarding serving coffee at a hot temperature. A customer sued Starbucks in federal court in Manhattan because she suffered third-degree burns on her ankle as a result of the company's steamy beverage (Enghagen & Gilardi, 2002). Just like many other cases, the result of this case is unknown due to lack of media coverage. It could have been settled, dismissed, or confidentially settled.

Again, at first glance, these cases may seem "frivolous." After looking further into the laws, case proceedings, and events of the incidents, these cases have merit and deserve proper evaluation by the jury, judge, and the public. It is important that criteria of the laws at hand are carefully examined from both sides. This is done to ensure that there is no doubt whether or not the plaintiff owes the defendant the amount in question. Liebeck vs McDonald's and Pearson vs Chungs are seemingly frivolous cases but do have some legal merit.

Epilogue

The best of authors have been known to write their work while in a drug-induced state. Alcohol is the most common drug of choice; however, cocaine is rather prevalent too. Some believe that these drugs contribute to an author's artistic abilities, while others believe it's just a coping mechanism for dealing with life's problems. Stephen King admitted he didn't remember writing "The Shining" (Miller, 2014). Coleridge wrote "Kubla Kahn" while high on opium. Poe was commonly found on the streets of Baltimore in a drunken stupor. Robert Louis Stevenson was an avid consumer of cocaine which gave him a super human writing stamina. He wrote his first draft of "Dr. Jekyll and Mr. Hyde", 30,000 words, in 3 days (Hossey, 2015). His wife hated the piece, so Stevenson snorted a few more lines and wrote his second draft, another 30,000 words, in 3 days. The most impressive thing about it was that this was in the days of writing with a feather quill.

Ayn Rand, the author of the longest and densest novels in the English language, wrote while under the influence of an amphetamine, legal equivalent of meth, in order to subdue her perfectionist tendencies. Voltaire was known to drink 50-70 cups of coffee a day which equates to one cup every ten minutes. Sartre, the philosopher that coined "existentialism", would take a daily barbiturate cocktail containing an average of 20 pills. The best of authors have been known to write their work while in a drug-induced state. This is by no means a justification, it is merely an observation.

Appendix A: Glossary

340B Prescription Drug Discount Program	The 340B Drug Discount Program is a U.S. federal government program created in 1992 under Section 340B of the Public Health Service Act and expanded under the Affordable Care Act that requires drug manufacturers to provide outpatient drugs to eligible healthcare organizations/ covered entities at significantly reduced prices.
ACA	See "Affordable Care Act"
Academic Detailing of Prescribers	Fact-based information about prescription drugs provided by credentialed clinicians to physicians and other prescribers. Traditional "detailing" refers to the process pharmaceutical manufacturer sales representatives use to promote their brand name drugs.

Accountable Care Organization (ACO)	A group of physicians, hospitals, and/or other providers who come together voluntarily and share the responsibility and financial risk of managing health delivery, costs, quality, and outcomes for groups of patients.
acquisition	when one company buys another or part of another company, or the company or part of a company that is bought
Actual Rebate Amount Per Script	Actual dollar amount of rebate for each prescription adjudicated. The amount may vary for retail and mail scripts.
ADD/ADHD	See "Attention Deficit Disorder/Attention Deficit Hyperactivity Disorder"
adherence	The patient's conformance with the healthcare provider's recommendation with respect to timing, dosage, and frequency of medication taken during the prescribed length of time.
Administrative Services Only (ASO)	An arrangement in which an organization funds its own employee benefit plan but hires an outside firm to perform specific administrative services such as processing prescription drug claims.

Affordable Care Act (ACA) The landmark health reform legislation passed by the 11th Congress and signed into law by President Barack Obama in March of 2010. This legislation, also known as the Patient Protection and Affordable Care Act (PPACA) includes a long list of health-related provisions that began taking place in 2010.

alliance an agreement between two or more organizations to work together

AMP See "Average Manufacturer Price"

Annual Out-of-Pocket (OOP) Limit The cap on the total amount a plan member pays each year.

ASO See "Administrative Services Only"

ASP See "Average Sales Price"

asset something belonging to an individual or a business that has value or the power to earn money

asynchronous This word is used in the telecommunications and distance learning fields. It has a similar meaning in both fields. In telecommunications, it refers to an exchange of data at intermittent, or non-synchronized intervals between two devices. In the distance learning field, it refers to learning systems in which the instructor and students do not have to synchronize their presence.

Attention Deficit Disorder/ Attention Deficit Hyperactivity Disorder (ADD/ADHD)
one of the most common childhood disorders characterized by symptoms such as difficulty with focus and attention, difficulty controlling behavior, and hyperactivity

attribute
a characteristic, feature, or quality

Average Manufacturer Price (AMP)
Recently modified under the Affordable Care Act, the new definition is the average price paid to the manufacturer for the drug by wholesalers for drugs distributed to retail community pharmacies and by retail community pharmacies that purchase drugs directly from the manufacturer. Excluded from the calculation of AMP are payments and rebates or discounts provided to certain providers and payers.

Average Sales Price (ASP)
ASP is determined using manufacturers' sales reports, which include information on total units sold and total revenue for each drug, and is subject to audit by Medicare.

Average Wholesale Price (AWP) A list-price benchmark for many pharmaceutical transactions that was created in the 1960's although there is no formal national legislative definition of AWP. Despite its name, the AWP does not represent actual marketplace transactions and does not accurately measure average prices from wholesalers to pharmacies.

AWP Discount (AWP Minus %) The negotiated amount a drug plan pays to pharmacies for the ingredient cost of a prescription, commonly expressed as a percentage off AWP.

balance sheet A document showing a company's financial position and wealth at a particular time. The balance sheet is often described as a 'photograph' of a company's financial situation at a particular moment.

benchmark 1 something that can be used as a comparison to judge or measure other things 2 good performance in a particular activity in one company that can be used as a standard to judge the s activity in other companies

beneficiary See "Member"

Biologic/Biotech Products

Includes a wide range of products such as vaccines, blood and blood components, allergens, somatic cells, gene therapy, tissues, and recombinant therapeutic proteins. Biologics are isolated from natural sources (human, animal, or microorganism). A subset of these products are typically called specialty drugs.

bits per second (bps)

This measures how much data can be transferred across a network connection. A bit is the smallest unit of information that computers deal with. Today we usually measure bps in kilobits per second or megabits per second. A kilobit is 1,000 bits, and a megabit is 1,000,000 bits.

brand drug

A brand name drug is a drug marketed under a proprietary, trademark-protected name.

bribery

dishonestly giving money to someone to persuade them to do something to help you

broker

a person or organization whose job is to buy and sell shares, currencies, property, insurance etc. for others

brown bagging   An alternative to the buy-and-bill process where drugs are dispensed by a specialty pharmacy directly to the patient who assumes responsibility for transporting the drugs to their healthcare provider's office for administration. Unlike buy-and-bill, the provider does not purchase the drug or seek drug reimbursement.

browser   A browser is also called a Web browser, because it is used to browse the content of the World Wide Web. The most popular browsers are Microsoft's Internet Explorer, Mozilla Firefox, Google Chrome, and Apple Safari. GUI browsers can display text, images, digital movies, sound, and other multimedia content. The original Web browsers could only display text.

bureaucracy   1 a system of governing that has a large number of departments and officials 2 disapproving all the complicated rules and processes of an official system, especially when they are confusing or responsible for causing a delay

Buy-and-Bill   Process for provider-administered outpatient drugs in which the health-care provider purchases, stores, and then administers the product to a patient. After the patient receives the drug and any other medical care, the provider submits a claim for reimbursement to the patient's insurer directly for the drug (using J-codes) and drug administration fees.

buyout   1 the act of buying a business 2 the act of buying all the shares in a company of a particular shareholder

C-DUR   See "Concurrent Drug Utilization Review"

Cadillac Tax   Under the Affordable Care Act, a 40% excise tax assessed on the cost of coverage for health plans considered to have very generous benefits that exceed a certain annual limit. The tax has been delayed from 2018 until 2020 by the Consolidated Appropriations Act of 2016.

capitation   A per member, monthly payment to a provider that covers contracted services to a defined population and paid in advance of service delivery.

Carve-In Pharmacy Benefit
Management of the drug benefit is included with the management of the medical benefit, using a single entity and contract to administer both benefits.

Carve-Out Pharmacy Benefit
Management of the drug benefit that is separate from the management of the medical benefit, using two different entities or two separate contracts to administer the benefits.

cash flow
1 the amounts of money coming into and going out of a company, and the timing of these 2 profit for a particular period, defined in different ways by different businesses

CDHP
See "Consumer-Directed Health Plan"

Centers for Medicare and Medicaid Services (CMS)
CMS provides oversight of the following federally funded healthcare programs: Medicare, Medicaid, the State Children's Health Insurance Program, and the Health Insurance Marketplace.

channel
Type of healthcare provider that may dispense a medication to a patient, including retail (community) pharmacy, mail service pharmacy, specialty pharmacy, infusion pharmacy, and medical provider (e.g., physician, hospital).

claim cost
See "Gross Cost of Script"

clipboard　An area of computer memory set aside for storing temporary copies of text, images, or other information, so that information can be copied from one document to another.

cloud computing　Computing that relies on networked storage or web applications is referred to as cloud computing. The name comes from the cloud shape traditionally used in network diagrams to refer to the Internet or another large network. Gmail and other Google Apps are an example of cloud computing.

CMS　See "Centers for Medicare and Medicaid Services"

coinsurance　A type of cost-sharing design in which the member pays a percentage share of the cost of a prescription; sometimes combined with "min/max" provisions for minimum or maximum out-of-pocket amounts; for example, a 20% coinsurance with a minimum of $20 and maximum of $100 per prescription.

competitive advantage　something that helps you to be better or more successful than others

compliance   Patient adherence to a prescribed
                          medical treatment plan or drug regi-
                          men.

compounded   Creation of personalized medica-
medications   tions for patients by a compound-
                          ing pharmacist who mixes together
                          individual ingredients to the exact
                          strength and dosage required by
                          the patient.

concept   an idea for a product, business etc.

Concurrent Drug   A drug utilization review performed
Utilization Review   during the course of treatment and
(C-DUR)   involves the ongoing monitoring
                          of drug therapy to ensure positive
                          patient outcomes. C-DUR presents
                          pharmacists with the opportunity to
                          alert prescribers to potential prob-
                          lems and to intervene in areas such
                          as drug-drug interactions, duplicate
                          therapy, over or underutilization,
                          and excessive or insufficient dosing.

conman   someone who tries to get money
                          from people by tricking them

consortium   a combination of several companies
                          working together for a particular
                          purpose, for example in order to
                          buy something or build something

consumer behavior the study of how, why, where, and when consumers buy things

Consumer-Directed Health Plan (CDHP) A high-deductible plan that is accompanied either by a health reimbursement arrangement (HRA) or is eligible for a health savings account (HSA). CDHPs encourage members to make informed decisions and spend their healthcare dollars wisely.

controlling interest the situation where one shareholder owns enough shares to control a company

copay A form of cost sharing where a portion of the prescription drug cost is paid by the member. Copays often vary based on product classification such as brand vs. generic or preferred vs. nonpreferred. The copay is kept by the pharmacy as part of the negotiated rate with the PBM. The copay is deducted from the total negotiated amount paid to the pharmacy by the PBM.

Copay Assistance Programs Pharmaceutical manufacturer-sponsored programs (also called copay coupon or copay offset programs) for branded drug products directed at the commercially insured patient population. These programs cover (offset) all or part of the drug copay up to a specified amount. Certain restrictions and eligibility requirements apply (for instance, not allowed for those with Medicare or Medicaid coverage).

Copayment Relief or Waivers   Reduced or zero-dollar copayments commonly used as incentives for plan members to use generic drugs and adhere to medication regimens.

corruption   1 the crime of giving or receiving money, gifts, a better job etc. in exchange for doing something dishonest or illegal that helps another person or company 2 when someone who has power or authority uses it in a dishonest or illegal way to get money or an advantage

cost sharing   Cost sharing refers to the amount members contribute to the cost of each prescription covered by their drug benefit plan. A cost share amount is established in the plan design for major categories of drugs such as brand, generic, or formulary classification. The amount may be a flat-dollar amount or a percentage of the total cost of the prescription.

Covered Entity   Covered entities are defined in the HIPAA rules as health plans, healthcare clearinghouses, and any healthcare provider, organization or corporation that directly handles Personal Health Information (PHI) or Personal Health Records (PHR), or who electronically transmits any health information in connection with transactions for which the Department of Health and Human Services (HHS) has adopted standards. The most common examples of covered entities include hospitals, doctors' offices, and health insurance providers.

crises   1 a period or moment of great difficulty, danger, or uncertainty, especially in politics or economics 2 a time when a personal problem or situation has reached its worst point

culture   1 the ideas, beliefs, and customs that are shared and accepted by people in a society 2 the attitudes or beliefs that are shared by a particular group of people or in a particular organization

customs   the government department responsible for collecting the tax on goods that have been brought into the country and making sure that illegal goods are not imported or exported

data warehouse A data warehouse is a database that is structured for reporting and querying. Data warehouses extract information from a variety of sources, including transactional database systems, clean and transform that data, then load it into a series of fact tables and dimension tables. The front end of the data warehouse provides end users with access to the data through pre-defined reports or tools that enable advanced users to slice and dice the data in many ways.

DAW See "Dispense as Written"

deductible Amount that a plan member pays out-of-pocket before benefit coverage begins.

defect a fault or the lack of something that means that a product etc. is not perfect

demand 1 spending on goods and services by companies and people in a particular economy 2 the total amount of a type of goods or services that people or companies buy in a particular period 3 the total amount of a type of goods or services that or companies would buy if they were available

deregulate
if a government deregulates a particular business activity, it allows companies to operate more freely so as to increase competition

detailing
The process pharmaceutical manufacturer sales representatives use to promote their brand-name drugs to prescribing physicians, nurse practitioners, and physician assistants.

diabetic supplies
Medical materials used in the treatment of diabetes, specifically glucose meter strips, syringes, and needles.

differentiation
when a company shows how its products are different from each other and from competing products, for example in its advertising

disclosure
1 the duty of someone in a professional position to inform customers, shareholders etc. about facts that will influence their decisions 2 the act of giving information about someone by an organization or person who would normally have to keep that information secret, for example when a bank gives information about a customer's accounts

to the police 3 a fact which is made known after being kept secret

Disease Management
A systematic approach to providing care to a population of patients with a specific disease. Patient and provider education, pharmaceutical care, continuous quality improvement, practice guidelines, patient monitoring, outcomes assessment, and case management may be included; however, program features vary widely.

Dispense as Written (DAW)
An order on a prescription indicating that the pharmacist should provide the patient with the prescription exactly as it was written. This is often used for a brand-name drug for which generic alternatives are available but the prescriber does not want a generic substituted.

Dispensing Fee
Contracted amount in a traditional third-party prescription plan that is paid to the pharmacy in addition to the negotiated ingredient cost of the prescription.

diversify
1 if a company or economy diversifies, it increases the range of goods or services it produces 2 to start to

put your money into different types of investments in addition to the investments you already have

DME See "Durable Medical Equipment"

DNS See "Domain Name System"

Dollar Limit on Coverage Price cap for amount of money plan will pay for prescription benefit.

Domain Name System (DNS) Domain Name System, a distributed database that maps computer hostnames to IP addresses. Computers that access the Internet need to be configured with the addresses of one or more DNS servers. Most computers receive their DNS server addresses through DHCP (Dynamic Host Configuration Protocol), the protocol used to automatically assign computers an IP address, subnet mask, and default gateway.

dose optimization Pharmacist-driven program to ensure patients are taking the best dosages and strengths of a given medication to manage costs of drug therapy.

drug benefit design Group of features that determine coverage terms, such as cost-sharing amounts, and utilization management requirements (e.g., prior authorization, step therapy).

Drug Utilization Review (DUR) — The process of evaluating prescribing patterns, and/or patient drug utilization against predetermined standards (e.g., treatment guidelines) to determine the appropriateness of drug therapy. Sometimes called drug use evaluation (DUE). There are three types: prospective (before prescription dispensing), concurrent (at point of dispensing), and retrospective (after a prescription is filled).

Durable Medical Equipment (DME) — Any equipment used to provide therapeutic benefits to a patient due to a specific medical condition(s). This equipment may include wheelchairs, crutches, walkers, monitors, etc.

economies of scale — the advantages that a bigger factory, shop etc. has over a smaller one because it can spread its fixed costs over a larger number of units and thus produce or sell things more cheaply

Employer Group Waiver Plan (EGWP) — Commonly referred to in retiree benefit plan parlance as an "egg whip", is a group Medicare Part D prescription drug plan option that is offered to retirees who have been promised prescription drug coverage as part of their Other Post-Employment Benefits (OPEB).

encryption

Encryption is the process of encoding information to prevent it from being read by unauthorized individuals. Human beings have been encrypting documents for centuries. In the 20th Century, nations and organizations began to use mechanical methods to improve their encryption methods; e.g., the German Enigma machine. In response, cryptanalysts (people who study and break encryption schemes) developed early computers to help them break the codes. Since that time, computer scientists and mathematicians have developed encryption methods based on a public/private key algorithm. These methods enable secure online communications for a variety of applications, such as electronic commerce, remote computer access, and email.

endorse

If someone, usually famous, endorses a product, they say how good it is in advertisements. People will buy the product because they like or trust the person.

Ethernet

Ethernet is a telecommunications protocol. We use it to connect computers to the local area network in our schools.

ethics

moral rules or principles of behavior that should guide members of a profession or organization and make them deal honestly and fairly with each other and with their customers

expand

1 to become larger in size, amount, or number, or to make something larger in size, amount, or number 2 if a company expands, it increases its sales, areas of activity etc.

experimental/in-vestigational drugs

Prescription drugs being tested in clinical trials; may or may not be approved for sale by the U.S. Food and Drug Administration (FDA).

FDB

See "First DataBank"

File Transfer Protocol (FTP)

This technology is used to transfer files between computers that are running the TCP/IP protocol suite. When you download a file from the Internet, you may use ftp. The most common type of ftp service is called anonymous ftp. This enables anyone to download files from an ftp server.

Firewall

In a building, a firewall is a wall that is used to contain the damage caused by a fire. In computing, a firewall is software or hardware that is used to contain the potential damage that can result from connecting your computer network to a public network, such as the Internet. Hackers and crackers use the Internet to attempt to break into private computer networks that are connected to the Internet.

First DataBank (FDB)

A commonly used database of pharmaceutical pricing information and clinical content used in the drug benefit industry.

focus group

A group of people brought together to discuss their feelings and opinions about a particular subject. In market research, focus groups discuss their opinions of products, advertisements, companies etc.

formulary

List of drugs used to treat patients in a drug benefit plan. Products listed on a formulary are covered for reimbursement at varying levels. The most common types of formulary are:

- Closed formulary: Nonformulary products are not covered for reimbursement in the benefit.
- Incented formulary: Formulary products are classified for reimbursement by product type including brand, generic, specialty, lifestyle, preferred, and nonpreferred.- -
- Incented formularies are increasingly popular because, when aligned with rational cost sharing levels, they help drive utilization to the lowest net cost drugs.
- Open formulary: Nonformulary products are covered at a defined level in the benefit.

franchise   1 an arrangement in which a company gives a business the right to sell its goods or services in return for payment or a share of the profits 2 a particular shop, restaurant etc. that is run under a franchise, or a company that owns a number of these franchise

Fraud, Waste, and Abuse (FWA)	Terminology that is used to describe intentional misrepresentation (fraud), overutilization or inappropriate utilization (waste), and inconsistent practices with respect to recognized standards of care for healthcare services resulting in additional costs.
FTP	See "File Transfer Protocol"
Fully-insured Plan	A plan that delegates financial risk of benefit claims to a third party.
Gb	See "gigabit"
GB	See "gigabyte"
GDP	See "Gross Domestic Product"
generic drug	A product that is comparable to a brand-name drug in dosage form, strength, route of administration, quality, performance characteristics, and intended use. Generics are typically less expensive and sold under the chemical name for the drug, not the brand name.
Generic Product Identifier (GPI)	A 14-character hierarchical classification system that identifies drugs from their primary therapeutic use down to the unique interchangeable product regardless of manufacturer or package size.

Generic Substitution The dispensing of the generic or multi-source product in place of the original brand-name drug. Most drug benefit plans mandate or in-cent generic substitution as a cost control mechanism. The U.S. Food and Drug Administration approves generic products. Generics with an "A" rating usually can be substituted for the brand product by the pharma-cist without contacting the physician.

GIF See "Graphics Interchange Format"

gigabit (Gb) A billion bits. New computers have network interface cards capable of transmitting and receiving data at one gigabit per second.

gigabyte (GB) A billion bytes. Please refer to the discussion of kilobits and kilobytes for clarification.

globalization the tendency for the world economy to work as one unit, led by large in-ternational companies doing busi-ness all over the world

GPI See "Generic Product Identifier"

Graphics Interchange Format (GIF) GIF is one of the three most com-mon graphics files formats used on the Internet. (JPEG and PNG are the others.) Internet browsers can display GIF files without any plug-ins or helper applications. The maximum number of colors that can be used in a GIF file is 256. This makes them best suited for drawings, charts, and other images which have large areas of flat color and distinct boundaries between colors. The JPEG format is better suited for full-color photographs. GIF and JPEG both use compression techniques to reduce the file size of the graphics they store. GIF uses lossless compression. GIF stands for Graphics Interchange Format.

Gross Cost of Script (Prescription) — Total cost of a prescription = AWP − AWP Discount + Dispensing Fee

Gross Domestic Product (GDP) — the total value of goods and services produced in a country's economy, not including income from abroad

gross domestic product per capital — the total value of goods and services produced in a country divided by the number of people living there

Guaranteed Rebate per Mail Script — Flat-dollar amount of a rebate guaranteed by a pharmacy benefit manager for each mail service prescription.

Guaranteed Rebate per Retail Script

Flat-dollar amount of a rebate guaranteed by a pharmacy benefit manager for each retail prescription.

Hacker

In the early days of computing, calling someone a hacker was a compliment. A hacker was someone who thoroughly understood how computers worked and was able to make them do all sorts of things that they may not have been designed to do. An elegant pieceof programming was called a hack. Today, hackers are thought of as outlaws: computer users who try to break into other people's computers. See cracker.

Health Insurance Portability and Accountability Act (HIPAA)

Enacted August 21, 1996, this United States law was designed to provide privacy standards to protect patients' medical records and other health information provided to health plans, doctors, hospitals, and other healthcare providers.

Hypertext Markup Language (HTML)

HTML consists of a set of tags for formatting World Wide Web pages. The tags control how your browser displays the page. For example, the text you are reading now is a definition. It is enclosed by <dd> and </dd> tags. A browser usually displays definition text by indenting it slightly from the left margin. Other tags are more complex.

Hypertext Transfer Protocol (HTTP) HTTP is the protocol upon which the World Wide Web is built. Tim Berners-Lee developed HTTP in the late 1980s to enable scientists to publish and share hypertext documents.

IDN See "Integrated Delivery Networks"

immersive photography Imagine you could take a photograph that includes a complete 360° field of view. This is the field of view that teachers who have eyes in the back of their heads see. Wrap that photograph around a transparent cylinder. Now imagine that you could shrink yourself and stand inside that cylinder. As you turn around, you would see the 360° scene from the same position as the photographer who made the picture. That is immersive photography. Apple Computer was the first company to demonstrate this, using QuickTimeVR® technology.

industrial espionage the activity of secretly finding out a company's plans, details of its products etc.

infant
An industry in its early stages of development in a particular country. Some people think that infant industries should be helped with government money and protected from international competition by import taxes etc.

infrastructure
1 the basic systems and structures that a country needs to make economic activity possible, for example transport, communications, and power supplies 2 the basic systems and equipment needed for an industry or business to operate successfully or for an activity to happen

Ingredient Cost
The component of a prescription drug claim cost that represents the cost of the medication; usually negotiated at a discount based on a pricing benchmark.

Injectable
Prescription drugs that are injected by the patient or the provider.

innovative
1 an innovative product, method, process etc. is new, different, and better than those that existed before 2 using clever new ideas and methods

Integrated Delivery Networks (IDN)
A network of site of care facilities and providers that work together to offer healthcare services to patients in a particular geographic area or market.

integrity
1 the state of being united or kept together as one whole, and therefore strong, unit 2 complete honesty

Java
An object-oriented computer programming language developed by Sun Microsystems. People are excited about Java because it represents a platform-independent language. In theory, you can write a program in Java and run it on a Linux, Macintosh, Unix, or Windows computer. The key to this platform independence is that Java programs run in what Sun calls a Java Virtual Machine, or JVM. Once a computer manufacturer writes a JVM for its computers, in theory any Java program could run on that JVM.

JavaScript
A computer scripting language that is most frequently used for adding interactivity to Web pages and validating data entry on web forms prior to their submission.

Joint Photographic Experts Group (JPEG)

JPEG is one of the three most common graphics files formats used on the Internet. (GIF and PNG are the others.) Internet browsers can display JPEG files without any plug-ins or helper applications. JPEG files are best suited for full-color images. JPEG uses a lossy compression method to reduce the size of the images it stores. (Lossy means that the compression technique works by discarding some of the information in the picture. JPEG technology allows for variable compressions schemes; that is, you can achieve smaller file sizes by using more compression, at the expense of picture quality.

joint venture

a business activity in which two or more companies have invested together

JQuery

A library of JavaScript functions. The JQuery library simplifies web application development by making available a large number of commonly used functions for purposes such as animation and event handling in a single, compact JavaScript file.

kilobit (kb)   A kilobit is 1,000 bits.

kilobyte (KB)   A kilobyte is 1,024 bytes. Why is a kilobit 1,000 bits and a kilobyte 1,024 bytes? The prefix kilo means 1,000, so a kilogram is 1,000 grams, and a kilometer is 1,000 meters, and a kilobit is 1,000 bits. In computer science, the term kilobit is used as a measure of network bandwidth. The term kilobyte is used as a measure of storage.

knowledge worker   someone whose job involves dealing with information, rather than making things

labor union   An organization representing people working in a particular industry or profession, especially in meetings with their employers.

laissez-faire   the idea that governments should do as little to the economy as possible and allow private business to develop without the state controlling or influencing them

LAMP   See "Linux-Apache-MySQL-PHP"

legend drug   Drug that, by law, can be obtained only by prescription and bears the label, "Caution: Federal law prohibits dispensing without a prescription" or "Rx Only."

letter of credit in foreign trade, a written promise by an importer's bank to pay the exporter's bank on a particular date or after a particular event, for example when the goods are sent by the exporter

liability 1 an amount of money owed by a business to a supplier, lender, or other creditor 2 liabilities the amounts of money owed by a business considered together, as shown in its balance sheet 3 a person's or organization's responsibility for loss, damage, or injury caused to others or their property, or for payment of debts

liberalize to make a system, laws, or moral attitudes less strict

lifestyle drugs Drugs that are not medically necessary but used to improve the quality of life.

limited company also limited liability company, a company where individual shareholders lose only the cost of their shares if the company goes bankrupt, and not other property they own

limited distribution pharmacy A pharmacy that has been contracted under a restricted network to distribute specialty medications to treat rare diseases.

limited pharmacy network
In a limited network, prescriptions are covered only in a subset of stores, typically by eliminating at least one major pharmacy chain from the network.

Linux-Apache-MySQL-PHP (LAMP)
A LAMP system is a computer running the Linux operating system, the Apache web server, the MySQL relational database management system, and the PHP (or Python or Perl) programming language interpreter. These four open-source applications provide an inexpensive, robust, and high-performance platform for developing web applications.

logo
a design or way of writing that a company or organization uses as its official sign on its products, advertising etc.

loophole
a small mistake in a law that makes it possible to do something the law is supposed to prevent you from doing, or to avoid doing something that the law is supposed to make you do

MAB
See "Maximum Allowable Benefit"

MAC
See "Maximum Allowable Cost"

MAC List   A list of drug products that are generally available with a generic version, to which MAC pricing will be applied. Both pricing and scope (i.e., number of drugs covered) of MAC lists may vary considerably by PBM and sometimes among customers of the same PBM.

mail service cost share   Cost share amount for a defined days-supply of a prescription therapy typically dispensed at a mail-service pharmacy. The amount may be a flat-dollar amount or a percentage of the total cost of the prescription.

mail service pharmacy   Licensed pharmacy established to dispense maintenance medications for chronic use in quantities greater than normally purchased at a retail pharmacy. The mail-service pharmacy usually uses highly automated equipment so that non-pharmacists perform many routine tasks. As a result, mail service can typically dispense medication at a lower cost per prescription.

maintenance medications   Drugs used to treat chronic diseases or conditions, such as diabetes, hypertension, and high cholesterol.

managed care   An organized system of healthcare delivery and monitoring intended to increase the cost-effectiveness of care while maintaining or increasing the quality of care; usually includes provider network management, measurement of health outcomes, and targeting of healthcare services to patients likely to benefit from them.

margin   also profit margin the difference between the price of a product or service and the cost of producing it, or between the cost of producing all of a company's products or services and the total sum they are sold for

market challenger   an organization or product that may take the place of the organization or product that has the highest sales in its market or industry

market leader   an organization or product that has the highest sales, or one of the highest sales, in its market or industry

Maximum Allowable Cost (MAC)   A pharmacy reimbursement limit for a particular strength and dosage of a generic drug that is available from multiple manufacturers with potentially different list prices. The MAC is established by the PBM or payer. The same MAC price applies to all versions of the identical generic drugs. MAC prices were created because the cost of identical generic drugs may differ from distributor to distributor.

Maximum Annual Benefit (MAB) Total amount of expenses a plan will pay in a 12-month period

Maximum Out of Pocket (MOOP) The most a covered member will pay for healthcare services. When this maximum has been reached, the member's healthcare plan pays 100 percent of the allowed amount for covered services.

Medi-Span A commonly used database of pharmaceutical pricing information and clinical content used in the drug benefit industry. Medi-Span is published by Wolters Kluwer. Wolters Kluwer also publishes Facts & Comparisons, a frequently used clinical reference for pharmacists.

Medication Therapy Management (MTM) A pharmacist-provided service that includes: 1 complete review of all medications, including herbals and over-the-counter products; 2 personal medication record (e.g., drugs, instructions, prescribers, allergies, problems); 3 medication action plan for the patient; 4 intervention and/ or referral to other healthcare providers; and 5 documentation. Previously known as "pharmaceutical care."

megabit (Mb) A megabit is one million bits.

megabyte (MB) A megabyte is 1,048,576 bytes (1,024 x 1,024). Please refer to the discussion of kilobits and kilobytes for clarification.

member A person who is covered by a prescription drug plan; alternatively described as an "enrollee" or "beneficiary."

middleman a person, business, organization etc. that buys things in order to sell them to someone else, or that helps to arrange business deals for other people

mission statement a short written statement made by an organization, intended to communicate its aims to customers, employees, shareholders etc.

model 1 a particular type or design of a vehicle or machine 2 a simple description or structure that is used to help people understand similar systems or structures 3 the way in which something is done by a particular country, person etc. that can be copied by others who want similar results

MOOP	See "Maximum Out of Pocket"
morale	the level of confidence and positive feelings among a group of people who work together
Moving Picture Experts Group Layer-3 (MP3)	A patented format used to encode compressed digital audio. The term is commonly used to refer to songs that have been encoded in this format. The MP3 format enables an uncompressed digital audio file to be significant reduced in size, at the loss of some audio quality.
MTM	See "Medication Therapy Management"
multi-source brand	A drug product manufactured by more than one company or source. Multi-source is commonly used to describe a brand drug where generic equivalents are available.
multi-tier copay	A cost-sharing structure with three or more categories or tiers of copay. The lowest copays are for generics, with increased amounts for the remaining categories.
narrow network	Benefit design that encourages or mandates use of particular retail pharmacies, such as restricting prescription fills to one or two retail pharmacy chains, or charging lower

copays at certain pharmacies. Used by plan sponsors and/or PBMs to obtain better pricing terms in exchange for higher prescription volume. The most common types of narrow networks are preferred pharmacy networks and limited networks.

National Drug Code (NDC) Numeric system to identify drug products in the United States. A drug's NDC number is often expressed using eleven digits in a 5-4-2 format (xxxxx-yyyy-zz) where the first five digits identify the manufacturer, the second four digits identify the product and strength, and the last two digits identify the package size and type.

National Institute for Health and Care Excellence (NICE) An institute that provides national guidance and advice to improve health and social care.

nepotism the practice of giving jobs to members of your family when you are in a position of power

net An abbreviation for network.

Net Cost of Script Gross cost minus the member cost-sharing amount. This is not necessarily the plan sponsors net cost as rebates are excluded from this calculation.

network
A group of computers, printers, and other devices that are connected together to exchange information. When used as a verb, network means the act of joining computers, printers, and other devices together; or the act of joining a computer to an existing network.

niche market
a market for a product or service, perhaps an expensive or unusual one that does not have many buyers but that may be profitable for companies who sell it

nonformulary drugs
Drugs not included on a plan's drug list or formulary.

nonpreferred brands
Brand-name drugs not included on a plan's preferred drug list.

on-site pharmacy
A no-owned pharmacy conveniently located on an employer or a healthcare company's site allowing access to needed medications to employees.

online adjudication
Electronic process of prescription drug claims at the point of service to verify coverage and detect potential problems that should be addressed before drugs are dispensed to patients.

Open Database Connectivity (ODBC)

Open Database Connectivity, a standard software interface for accessing database management systems, such as Oracle, SQL Server, or MySQL.

open source

Software of which the source code is free available to the general public. Open source software is also available to freely download and use.

Optical Character Recognition (OCR)

OCR software is capable of converting a digital image of a page of scanned text into editable text. The degree of accuracy varies with the quality of the original text.

optical drive

A CD-ROM drive, DVD drive, or other device that uses a laser to record and/or write data onto an optical disk. Read-only and ready-write optical drives have been the workhorses of removable data storage for a number of years, but are gradually being supplanted by USB drives and cloud-based storage.

optimize

to make the best possible use of something or to do something in the best possible way

oral contraceptives

Oral prescription drugs used to avoid pregnancy.

Orange Book Authoritative source on therapeutic equivalence ratings of drug products approved by the U.S. Food and Drug Administration (FDA). The official name is the FDA's Approved Drug Products with Therapeutic Equivalence Evaluations. The common name, Orange Book, is a result of the original color of the book's cover.

orphan drug A pharmaceutical agent that has been developed specifically to treat a rare medical condition; the condition itself being referred to as an orphan disease.

Out-of-Pocket (OOP) Costs Patient paid portion of prescription costs, typically in the form of copays or coinsurance.

Over-the-Counter (OTC) Drug U.S. Food and Drug Administration (FDA)-approved drugs that do not require a prescription to be purchased.

P&T See "Pharmacy and Therapeutics Committee"

PA See "Prior Authorization"

pass-thru pricing An arrangement in which a plan sponsor pays the exact amount paid to the pharmacy (i.e., no mark-up).

patent	a legal document giving a person or company the right to make or sell a new invention, product, or method of doing something and stating that no other person or company is allowed to do this
Patient Assistance Programs (PAPs)	Assistance offered by nonprofit organizations/ foundations and pharmaceutical manufacturers to help patients in need to access prescribed drug treatments. Typically these are intended for patients who are not insured or have demonstrated financial need. Eligibility criteria vary by program and are typically based on a percentage of the federal poverty level.
PBA	See "Pharmacy Benefit Administrator"
PBM	See "Pharmacy Benefit Manager"
PDP	See "Prescription Drug Plan"
Peer-to-Peer Network	A peer-to-peer network, usually abbreviated p2p, is a group of network nodes or devices that can share content with one another. Many file-sharing sites are implemented as p2p networks.

Per Member Per Month (PMPM) Measure used to assess population-based metrics such as cost or utilization, computed by dividing the total cost/utilization/other measure by the total number in the population.

persistency Obtaining prescribed refills of medication at regular, appropriate intervals.

petabyte 1,000,000 gigabytes. In the International System of Units (SI), peta means 1015, so 1 petabyte = 1,000,000,000,000,000 bytes. Some very large databases occupy multiple petabytes of disk space.

Pharmacogenomics The study of how genes affect a person's response to drugs. This field combines pharmacology (the science of drugs) and genomics (the study of genes and their functions) to develop effective, safe medications, and doses that will be tailored to a person's genetic makeup.

Pharmacy and Therapeutics (P&T) Committee Group of physicians, pharmacists, and other healthcare providers from different specialties who advise a pharmacy benefit manager, hospital, or managed care organization on the safe and effective use of medications. The P&T Committee manages the formulary, reviews new drugs to market to help determine formulary status, and establishes drug use guidelines and policies.

Pharmacy Benefit Administrator (PBA) Organization that supports the administrative and information system needs of prescription benefit programs. A PBA usually maintains eligibility, and processes and adjudicates prescription claims similar to what administrative services only (ASO) organizations do in the major medical arena.

Pharmacy Benefit Manager (PBM) Organization dedicated to administering prescription benefit management services to employers, health plans, third-party administrators, union groups, and other plan sponsors. A full-service PBM maintains eligibility, adjudicates prescription claims, provides clinical services and customer support, contracts and manages pharmacy networks, and provides management reports. PBMI provides a PBM Directory.

pill splitting   Cutting prescription medications in half to double the number of days' supply from one prescription, thereby decreasing the cost of the drug therapy.

pioneer   the first person or organization to do something that other people and organizations will later develop or continue to do

PMPM   See "Per Member Per Month"

Point of Sale (POS)   A drug store or pharmacy where a prescription can be filled and the medication is delivered to the member.

preferred brands   Brand-name drugs included on plan's preferred drug list.

preferred drug list   List of drugs that have been designated as preferred by a plan, usually based on formulary review of efficacy, safety, and cost considerations. These drugs are often made available to plan members at a lower cost-sharing amount than drugs considered nonpreferred.

preferred pharmacy network   In a preferred pharmacy network arrangement, consumers pay a lower out-of-pocket cost-sharing amount in certain stores and/or chains.

prescriber The licensed clinician – a physician, nurse practitioner, or physician assistant – who writes a prescription for a patient. The type of clinician who is legally allowed to prescribe varies by state because prescribing is governed by state law.

prescriber profiling Assessment of prescribing patterns to identify areas to manage utilization and cost of prescription drugs. Drug claim data is cut by prescriber (physician, physician assistant, or nurse practitioner) to identify outliers in prescribing patterns.

Prescription Drug Plan (PDP) U.S. Centers for Medicare & Medicaid Services certified drug benefit program for the Medicare eligible population.

price protection A ceiling or cap put on the amount a manufacturer can increase the cost of a medication during the life of the rebate contract with the PBM. Depending on client contract terms, additional savings may or may not be shared with the plan sponsor.

Prior Authorization (PA) A process under which a prescription claim is initially denied so that the health plan can evaluate the therapy

	before treatment starts. This process typically requires action from the physician, pharmacist, or patient to obtain coverage.
prototype	the first form that a new design of a car, machine etc. has
QL	See "Quantity Limits"
qualification	1 an examination that you have passed at school, university, or in your profession 2 a skill, personal quality, or type of experience that makes you suitable for a particular job
quality circle	a small group of employees who meet regularly to discuss ways to improve working methods and to solve problems
Quality of Service (QoS)	Quality of Service, a technology used to provide guaranteed bandwidth and priority for time-sensitive network applications, such as video conferencing.
Quantity Limits (QL)	A limit on the number of pills or dosages of a prescription drug that will be covered, either per claim or per unit of time (e.g., monthly).
quota	an official limit on the number or amount of something that is allowed in a particular period

R&D See "Research and Development"

R-DUR See "Retrospective Drug Utilization Review"

rationalize to make a business or organization more effective by getting rid of unnecessary staff, equipment etc, or reorganizing its structure

Rebate Amount per Script Dollar amount of a rebate for each prescription adjudicated. The amount may vary for retail and mail service scripts.

recall 1 if a company recalls one of its products, it asks customers to return it because there may be something wrong with it 2 to remember something that you have seen or heard, such as an advertisement

Red Book A commonly used database of pharmaceutical pricing information and clinical content used in the drug benefit industry. Red Book is published by Truven Health Analytics. This company also publishes Micromedex, a commonly used clinical reference database for pharmacists.

Reference-Based Pricing Setting of the reimbursement for a healthcare service at a maximum level or capped amount; the patient can choose a higher-priced service but must pay the difference between the actual cost and the reference price.

Refill-Too-Soon (RTS) Supply Limit
A system edit that rejects a drug claim if a refill is requested before a predefined number of days have passed since the last fill date of that prescription.

Relational Database Management System (RDBMS)
An RDBMS is software that manages relational databases; that is, databases that consist of a number of related tables that model some real-world system. RDBMS software enables users to create tables that can store millions of rows of information, enforce referential integrity rules on the information stored in those tables, and query the data stored in those tables.

reliable
someone or something that is reliable can be trusted or depended on

Research and Development (R&D)
the part of a business concerned with studying new ideas and developing new products

restriction
an official rule that limits or controls what people can do or what is allowed to happen

Retail Cost Share
Cost share amount for 30 days of a prescription therapy dispensed at a retail pharmacy. The amount may be

a flat-dollar amount or a percentage of the total cost of the prescription.

retailer 1 a business that sells goods to members of the public, rather than to shops etc. 2 someone who owns or runs a shop selling goods to members of the public

Retiree Drug Subsidy Amount of money the U.S. Centers for Medicare & Medicaid Services pays employers to subsidize employers' funding of drug benefits for Medicare eligible employees and retirees.

Retrospective Drug Utilization Review (R-DUR) Drug utilization review conducted after a prescription is adjudicated and the patient has received the medication. R-DUR may detect patterns in prescribing, dispensing, or administering drugs to prevent recurrence of inappropriate use or abuse and serves as a means for developing prospective standards and target interventions.

router A router is a specialized computer that connects local area networks to wide area networks.

scanner A device that converts a picture, printed text, a barcode, or some other physical form of information into a digital form that a computer can read. Scanners are commonly used to convert photographs into digital images.

search engine A Web site that enables users to search for Web pages by entering keywords. Yahoo was the first successful search engine. When you create a Web site, it does not automatically appear in a search engine's index. Most search engines enable you to add your site to their index, with your choice of keywords.

Self-insured Plan Plan that assumes financial risk for benefit claims.

sell-off when a business, company etc., or part of one, is sold to another company

single-source brand A drug product manufactured by one company or source.

Site of Care/Site of Service The various locations where patients can be treated, including hospital outpatient facilities, standalone infusion centers, physician offices, and patient homes. Drug treatment costs may vary across these sites, and reimbursement management of drugs and drug benefit designs often include site of care management to ensure that the highest value sites of services are utilized.

skill
an ability to do something well, especially because you have learned and practiced it

sleeping partner
a partner who invests in a business but does not take an active part in managing it

Specialty Drugs
Drugs that treat chronic, complex, or life-threatening conditions, usually manufactured through biologic processes and/or targeting a specific gene. Typically these medications are costly and require intensive clinical monitoring, complex patient actions, and/or special handling by the dispensing pharmacy.

specialty pharmacies
A channel to deliver specialty drugs directly to patients or healthcare providers. Specialty pharmacies are responsible for drug inventory, storage and handling, drug preparation, and billing the payer for the drug. They also monitor patient adherence and typically offer 24/7 patient support and education. Drug benefit design can require that patients

use a designated specialty pharmacy to obtain specific drugs. Some drug manufacturers also only distribute select drugs through an exclusive or limited number of designated specialty pharmacies.

specialty pharmacy benefit   Coverage of specialty drugs, often using different utilization management techniques (e.g., PA, step therapy) and cost-sharing amounts than are used for traditional medications.

Split-Fill Program   A method of dispensing intended to reduce drug waste due to patient intolerability where drugs known for high discontinuation rates upon initiation are initially dispensed for less than a full month supply (e.g., short fill for 1 week, 10 days, 2 weeks, etc.).

Spread Pricing   A type of contracting for PBM services in which the amount paid by the plan sponsor to the PBM for the prescription is greater than the amount paid by the PBM to the pharmacy.

stake   money risked or invested in a business

Step Therapy (ST)   Treatment guidelines used to recommend drug therapy beginning with a drug that is less expensive and/ or with which there is more post marketing safety experience. More expensive therapies are only used when the patient fails to respond to the first-line drug or after a PA.

streaming audio Streaming audio solves a problem that used to discourage the use of sound on the Internet. Before streaming audio, Web users had to download an entire sound file before they could hear it. Because sound files tend to be fairly large, users had to wait a long time before they could hear the file. Web browsers can begin playing streaming audio files a few seconds after the download begins. In other words, you hear the file *as it streams into your computer,* rather than after it arrives.

subliminal advertising when images appear very quickly during a television or cinema advertisement with effects that people are not conscious of

subsidy money that is paid by a government or organization to make something cheaper to buy, use, or produce

swindle to get money from someone dishonestly by deceiving them

tariff
a tax on goods coming into a country or going out of it

terabyte
1,000 gigabytes. In the International System of Units (SI), tera means 1012, so 1 terabyte = 1,000,000,000,000 bytes. Disk drives of 1 terabyte or larger have now become commonplace.

Therapeutic Substitution
A pharmacist-initiated change in a dispensed drug when a medically equivalent drug is available for the prescription presented. State prescribing laws address the required physician permission for substitutions.

Third Party Administrator (TPA)
Reseller of pharmacy benefit management services to small employer groups. TPAs can be full service, providing additional services such as dental, medical and vision, etc. They can be owned by a larger insurance carrier and they may specialize in pharmacy only or other specific areas.

tier
Category used to establish the member's cost sharing levels for medications, with generic drugs typically in Tier 1 (lowest cost-sharing) and brand drugs in higher tiers.

Total Quality Management (TQM) the management of systems in a company in order to make sure that each department is working in the most effective way and to improve the quality of the goods the company produces

TPA See "Third Party Administrator"

transaction 1 a business deal, especially one involving the exchange of money 2 the act of paying or receiving money

Transmission Control Protocol/ Internet Protocol (TCP/IP) The world's most popular computer networking protocol. TCP/IP is actually a suite of several different protocols: TCP, IP, FTP, HTTP, etc.

Transparency/ Transparent Pricing Full disclosure of all revenue streams including, formulary management fees, data sales, margin pricing, rebates etc., is made available.

treatment guidelines A comprehensive document designed to guide decisions and criteria regarding diagnosis, management, and treatment in specific areas of healthcare. These medical guidelines (also called clinical guidelines, clinical protocols, or clinical practice guidelines) are common in complex conditions such as cancer and represent recommended

	interventions based on high-level evidence and expert judgment.
UM	See "Utilization Management"
unique selling proposition	also unique selling point (USP) the thing that makes a particular product different from all other similar products
Usual and Customary (U&C) Price	Price charged to a cash-paying customer for a prescription product. Pharmacy benefit managers and health plans typically mandate that pharmacies accept reimbursement at the negotiated discount or the U&C price, whichever is lower. Payers should require that this be included in their PBM contracts to help manage costs.
Utilization Management (UM)	Utilization management is the process of evaluating the necessity, appropriateness, and efficiency of healthcare services against established guidelines and criteria. Common utilization management programs include prior authorization, step therapy, and quantity limits.
virtualization	The process of creating virtual machines, or guest computers that run entirely within virtualization

software. Server virtualization is a popular technology for reducing hardware and operating costs while increasing reliability and uptime. A common server virtualization configuration employs multiple servers running software called a hypervisor that enables the servers to host a number of virtual operating systems.

virus A malicious computer program that secretly installs itself on a computer or attaches itself to one or more files running on a host computer. Strictly speaking, a computer virus has the ability to copy itself and infect other computers across a network or through shared media, such as USB drives.

WAC See "Wholesale Acquisition Cost"

warranty A written promise that a company gives to a customer, stating that it will repair or replace a product they have bought if it breaks during a certain period of time. Warranty is another word for guarantee.

whistleblower someone working for an organization who tells the authorities that people in the are doing something illegal, dishonest, or wrong

White Bagging

An alternative to the buy-and-bill process where drugs are dispensed by a specialty pharmacy directly to the patient's healthcare provider for administration. Unlike buy-and-bill, the provider does not purchase the drug or seek drug reimbursement.

Wholesale Acquisition Cost (WAC)

Defined by statute as the pharmaceutical manufacturer's list price to wholesalers or direct purchasers in the United States.

wholesaler

a person or company that sells goods in large quantities to other businesses, who may then sell them to the general public

World Wide Web (WWW)

The World Wide Web is the most popular Internet information service. It is so popular that many Internet newcomers think that it *is* the Internet. It is, however, another Internet service like electronic mail and ftp. Ease of use made the World Wide Web popular, and the staggering amount of information available on it will ensure that its popularity increases.

Wrap Around Coverage

Drug benefit coverage provided by employers to Medicare-eligible employees and retirees to supplement Medicare Part D coverage.

Adapted from:

Drug Benefit Glossary: Common Drug Benefit Terminology. (2017) (1st ed.). Plano. Retrieved from https://www.pbmi. com/PBMI/Services/Drug_Benefit_Glossary/PBMI/ Services/Drug_Benefit_Glossary.aspx?hkey=1051faba-063f-4ae3-a95b-70cd0476f1db

Glossary of Business Terms. (2017) (1st ed.). Steinhausen. Retrieved from https://www.pearson.ch/download/ media/9781405881357_Glossary_ML_Int.pdf

Glossary of Technology Terms. (2017). *Smyth County School Board.* Retrieved from http://www.scsb.org/glossary. html

Appendix B: References

Adams, V. (2002). Randomized Controlled Crime: Postcolonial Sciences in Alternative Medicine Research. *Social Studies Of Science, 32*(5-6), 659-690. doi:10.1177/030631270203200503

Adokiya, M. N., Awoonor-Williams, J. K., Beiersmann, C., & Müller, O. (2016). Evaluation of the reporting completeness and timeliness of the integrated disease surveillance and response system in northern Ghana. *Ghana Medical Journal, 50*(1), 3-8.

Aguinis, H., Joo, H., & Gottfredson, R. (2011). Why we hate performance management - And why we should love it. *Business Horizons, 54*(6), 503-507. doi:10.1016/j.bushor.2011.06.001

Aguinis, H., Gottfredson, R., & Joo, H. (2012a). Delivering effective performance feedback: The strengths-based approach. *Business Horizons, 55*(2), 105-111. doi:10.1016/j.bushor.2011.10.004

Aguinis, H., Joo, H., & Gottfredson, R. (2012b). Performance management universals: Think globally and act locally. *Business Horizons, 55*(4), 385-392. doi:10.1016/j.bushor.2012.03.004

Alba, D. (2015). *The Chinese Ride-Hailing Startup That's Out-Ubering Uber. WIRED.* Retrieved from https://www.wired.com/2015/06/the-chinese-ride-hailing-startup-thats-out-ubering-uber/

Allemand, A. (2017). *Market-Driven Approaches to Managing the Rise in Drug Prices. Pharmacy Benefit Management Institute.* Lecture, Orlando, FL.

Allen, T. D., Golden, T. D., & Shockley, K. M. (2015). How Effective Is Telecommuting? Assessing the Status of Our Scientific Findings. *Psychological Science In The Public Interest (Sage Publications Inc.), 16*(2), 40-68. doi:10.1177/1529100615593273

Almquist, E., Senior, J., & Bloch, N. (2016). The Elements of Value. *Harvard Business Review.* Retrieved from https://hbr.org/2016/09/the-elements-of-value

Altstedter, A. & Trivedo, U. (2017). *Limiting A Drug's Use To Maintain Its Efficacy. Bloomberg Businessweek.* Retrieved from https://www.scribd.com/article/336402151/Limiting-A-Drug-S-Use-To-Maintain-Its-Efficacy

Amelinckx, A. (2011). *Law firm will screen film. The Berkshire Eagle.* Retrieved from http://www.berkshireeagle.com/stories/law-firm-will-screen-film,435044?

Ang, P. (2015). *How Countries Are Regulating Internet Content. Internet Society.* Retrieved from https://www. isoc.org/inet97/proceedings/B1/B1_3.HTM

Appleby, J. (2017). *How Medicare Drug Plans Hope To Follow Private Sector Lead. Kaiser Health News.* Retrieved from http://khn.org/news/how-medicare-drug-plans-hope-to-follow-private-sector-lead/

Balick, R. (2016). *DEA limits opioid controlled substances to be manufactured in 2017. Pharmacy Today.* Retrieved from http://pharmacytoday.org/article/S1042-0991(16)31407-4/fulltext

Barry, P. (2016). *Medicare Enrollment Mistakes. AARP.* Retrieved from http://www.aarp.org/health/health-insurance/info-2014/medicare-mistakes-to-avoid.html

Benamati, J., Fuller, M., Serva, M., & Baroudi, J. (2010). Clarifying the Integration of Trust and TAM in E-Commerce Environments: Implications for Systems Design and Management. *IEEE Transactions On Engineering Management, 57*(3), 380-393. doi:10.1109/tem.2009.2023111

Benedict, N. (2010). Virtual Patients and Problem-Based Learning in Advanced Therapeutics. *American Journal of Pharmaceutical Education, 74.* doi:10.5688/aj7408143

Bennett, C. (2001). Cookies, web bugs, webcams and cue cats: Patterns of surveillance on the world wide web. *Ethics And Information Technology, 3*, 197-210.

Bhattacharya, M., Shahrawat, R., & Joon, V. (2012). Understanding Level of Maternal and Child Health Indicators used in Health Management Information System among Peripheral Level Health Functionaries in Two Districts of India. *Journal Of Health Informatics In Developing Countries*, *6*(1), 385-395.

Bhattacherjee, A. (2002). Individual Trust in Online Firms: scale development and initial test. *Journal Of Management Information Systems*, *19*(1), 211-241.

Biddle, B. (1986). Recent Developments in Role Theory. *Annual Review Of Sociology*, *12*(1), 67-92. doi:10.1146/annurev.soc.12.1.67

Big Pharma Spends More On Advertising Than Research And Development, Study Finds. (2008). *ScienceDaily*. Retrieved from https://www.sciencedaily.com/releases/2008/01/080105140107.htm

Bolte, J. (2014). The big question about lean six sigma. *Industrial Engineer*, *46*(4), 50-53.

Bonner, L. (2017). Staying in the know about EpiPen alternatives in 2017. *Pharmacy Today*, *23*(1), 36. Retrieved from http://pharmacytoday.org/article/S1042-0991(16)31643-7/abstract

Borchgrevink, C., Susskind, A., & Tarras, J. (1998). Consumer preferred hot beverage temperatures. *Food Quality and Preference, 10*. Retrieved from https://scholars.opb.msu.edu/en/publications/consumer-preferred-hot-beverage-temperatures-2

Branson, L., Chen, L., & Redenbaugh, K. (2013). The Presence of Women in Top Executive Positions in Non-Profit Organizations and Fortune 500 Companies. *International Journal Of Business And Public Administration, 10*(2), 15-29.

Brodesser-Akner, T. (2016). *Even the World's Top Life Coaches Need a Life Coach. Meet Martha Beck. Bloomberg.* Retrieved from https://www.bloomberg.com/features/2016-martha-beck-life-coach/

Brodkin, J. (2009). Where Apple stands in the enterprise. *Network Week, 26*(2), 12-38.

Brody, L. (2016). Planet 2.0. *Forbes*, 82-88.

Brown, D., Brown, D., & Yocum, C. (2012). Planning a pharmacy-led medical mission trip, part 2: Servant leadership and team dynamics. *Annals Of Pharmacotherapy, 46*(6), 895-900. doi:10.1345/aph.1q547

Brown, E. (2016). *Is a copyright registration required before filing an infringement lawsuit?. Internet Cases.* Retrieved from http://blog.internetcases.com/

Brown, L. (2009). Measurement of pharmacy quality metrics at the pharmacy level should be our goal. *Journal of the American Pharmacists Association, 49*(2), 153. doi:10.1331/japha.2009.09030

Browning, J. (2011). Legally speaking: Separating myths from reality-the truth about 'hot coffee.' *Southeast Texas Record.* Retrieved from http://setexasrecord.com/

Business Email Compromise. (2015). *Internet Crime Complaint Center (IC3).* Retrieved from https://www.ic3.gov/media/2015/150827-1.aspx

Business Intelligence vs. Data Analytics. (2015). *CyberTrend.* Retrieved from https://www.cybertrend.com/article/17281/business-intelligence-vs-data-analytics

Business Technology News. (2017). *CyberTrend.* Retrieved from https://www.cybertrend.com/article/24254/business-technology-news

Caldwell, T. (2013). Spear-phishing: how to spot and mitigate the menace. *Computer Fraud & Security, 2013*(1), 11-16. doi:10.1016/s1361-3723(13)70007-1

Campbell, M. & Gretler, C. (2016). *Nestlé Wants to Sell You Both Sugary Snacks and Diabetes Pills. Bloomberg Businessweek.* Retrieved from https://www.bloomberg.com/news/features/2016-05-05/nestl-s-sugar-empire-is-on-a-health-kick

Canfield, B. & Schelin, L. (2017). *Using Technology to Drive Greater Member Engagement. Pharmacy Benefit Management Institute.* Lecture, Orlando, FL.

Cascio, W. (1982). Scientific, Legal, and Operational Imperatives of Workable Performance Appraisal Systems. *Public Personnel Management, 11*(4), 367-375.

Cascio, W. (2011). The Puzzle of Performance Management in the Multinational Enterprise. *Industrial And Organizational Psychology, 4*(2), 190-193. doi:10.1111/j.1754-9434.2011.01324.x

Cha, A. (2016). *Opioid pills 'are like guns': More than 13,000 children were poisoned during six-year period. The Washington Post.* Retrieved from https://www.washingtonpost.com/news/to-your-health/wp/2016/10/31/opioid-pills-like-guns-more-than-13000-children-were-poisoned-during-six-year-period/?utm_term=.cd-68b9acd438

Chafkin, M. (2016a). *IBM's First Female CEO Is Taking On The Future. Bloomberg Businessweek.* Retrieved from https://www.bloomberg.com/features/2016-ginni-rometty-interview-issue/

Chafkin, M. (2016b). *Uber Debuts Its First Fleet of Driverless Cars in Pittsburgh. Bloomberg Businessweek.* Retrieved from https://www.bloomberg.com/news/features/2016-08-18/uber-s-first-self-driving-fleet-arrives-in-pittsburgh-this-month-is06r7on

Chafkin, M. & Bergen, M. (2016). *Google Makes So Much Money, It Never Had to Worry About Financial Discipline - Until Now. Bloomberg.* Retrieved from https://www.bloomberg.com/news/features/2016-12-08/google-makes-so-much-money-it-never-had-to-worry-about-financial-discipline

China Focus: Avon bribery scandal bodes poorly for multinational companies. (2012). *Xinhua Economic News.* Retrieved from http://www.china.org.cn/business/2012-02/22/content_24698218.htm

Chiu, C., Lin, H., Sun, S., & Hsu, M. (2009). Understanding customers' loyalty intentions towards online shopping:

an integration of technology acceptance model and fairness theory. *Behaviour & Information Technology, 28*(4), 347-360. doi:10.1080/01449290801892492

Clark, S. (2014). A vision for the future of pharmacy residency training. *American Journal of Health-System Pharmacy, 71*, 1196-8. doi:10.2146/ajhp140113

Clark, T., Kokko, H., & White, S. (2012). Trust: An essential element of leaders and managers. *American Journal Of Health-System Pharmacy, 69*(11), 928-930. doi:10.2146/ajhp110516

Cognitive Computing Explained: AI, Natural Language Processing & Machine Learning User in a new era. (2017). *CyberTrend.* Retrieved from https://www.cybertrend.com/article/24264/cognitive-computing-explained

Coy, P. (2016). *The EpiPen Drama Shows What's Wrong With How Drugs Are Priced. Bloomberg Businessweek.* Retrieved from https://www.bloomberg.com/news/articles/2016-09-01/the-epipen-drama-shows-what-s-wrong-with-how-drugs-are-priced

Cryptocurrency Trader Launches Super Deal for Bitcoin Sellers. (2015). *MarketWired.* Retrieved from https://finance.yahoo.com/news/cryptocurrency-trader-launches-super-deal-220905912.html

Daniels, J., Radebaugh, L., & Sullivan, D. (2015). *International business* (15th ed.). Upper Saddle River, NJ: Pearson.

Dave, P. (2015). *IRS hack: What to do when your Social Security number is exposed. Los Angeles Times.* Retrieved from http://www.latimes.com/business/technology/la-fi-tn-irs-social-security-20150527-story.html

Desselle, S., Vaughan, M., & Faria, T. (2002). Creating a Performance Appraisal Template for Pharmacy Technicians Using the Method of Equal-Appearing Intervals. *Journal Of The American Pharmaceutical Association, 42*(5), 768-779. doi:10.1331/108658002764653540

DHIS 2 End-User Manual. 2nd ed. 2016. Web. 20 July 2016.

DHIS 2 In Action. DHIS2.org. 2016. Web. 31 June 2016.

Diffin, J., Chirombo, F., & Nangle, D. (2010). Cloud Collaboration: Using Microsoft SharePoint as a Tool to Enhance Access Services. *Journal Of Library Administration, 50*(5-6), 570-580. doi:10.1080/01930826.20 10.488619

Dirks, K., Kim, P., Ferrin, D., & Cooper, C. (2011). Understanding the effects of substantive responses on trust following a transgression. *Organizational Behavior and Human Decision Processes, 114*(2), 87-103. doi:10.1016/j.obhdp.2010.10.003

Drane, A. (2016). *What's Really Killing Us?. Quality Talks 2016.* Retrieved from http://www.qualitytalks.org/events/qt-2016/talks/whats-really-killing-us/

Eddy, N. (2009). *Netsuite Brings Cloud Computing ERP Suite to the iPhone. eWeek.* Retrieved from http://

www.eweek.com/enterprise-apps/netsuite-brings-cloud-computing-erp-suite-to-the-iphone

Elliott, C. (2010). *Making a Killing: Clinical trials have become marketing exercises for Big Pharma - and cash-strapped universities are helping make the sale. NARPA.* Retrieved from http://www.narpa.org/makingakilling.htm

Enghagen, L. & Gilardi, A. (2002). McDonald's and the $2.9 million cup of coffee: Putting things in perspective. *Cornell Hotel and Restaurant Administration Quarterly, 43.* doi:10.1177/0010880402433005

Eroding exceptionalism: Internet firms' legal immunity is under threat. (2017). *The Economist.* Retrieved from http://www.economist.com/news/business/21716661-platforms-have-benefited-greatly-special-legal-and-regulatory-treatment-internet-firms

Esserman, L. (2016). *Tailored Cancer Care: Less Can Be More. Quality Talks 2016.* Retrieved from http://www.qualitytalks.org/events/qt-2016/talks/tailored-cancer-care-less-can/

Farndale, E. & Kelliher, C. (2013). Implementing Performance Appraisal: Exploring the Employee Experience. *Human Resource Management, 52*(6), 879-897. doi:10.1002/hrm.21575

Flynn, S. (2015). Technology in Global Markets. *Research Starters: Business (Online Edition).*

Fox, J. (2016). *The Strange Case of Off-Patent Drug Price Gougers. Bloomberg View.* Retrieved from https://

www.bloomberg.com/view/articles/2016-09-09/the-strange-case-of-off-patent-drug-price-gougers

Francke, G. (1955). *How much we need leaders in hospital pharmacy!.* Lecture, Washington, D.C.

Fusilier, M. & Penrod, C. (2009). e-Crime Prevention: An Investigation of the Preparation of e-Commerce Professionals. *Journal Of Internet Commerce, 8*(1-2), 2-22. doi:10.1080/15332860903341281

Galli, B. & Handley, H. (2014). The right approach to six sigma leadership. *Industrial Management, 56*(3), 25-30.

Giddens, A. (1997). *Sociology, Third Edition.* Cambridge: Polity Press.

Ginni Rometty. (2017). *Forbes.* Retrieved from https://www.forbes.com/profile/ginni-rometty/

Goldratt, E. & Cox, J. (2012). *The Goal: A Process of Ongoing Improvement.* Great Barrington, MA: North River Press.

Goldstein, S. (2007). *$54 million pants suit does not have legs: A court rejected claims of a D.C. man who sued his dry cleaners. The Philadelphia Inquirer.* Retrieved from https://www.newspapers.com/newspage/199564118/

Goodall, N. (2016). *Can You Program Ethics Into a Self-Driving Car?. IEEE Spectrum.* Retrieved from http://spectrum.ieee.org/transportation/self-driving/can-you-program-ethics-into-a-selfdriving-car

Gottlieb, S. (2017). *What Lies Ahead? Perspectives on Healthcare Policy Reform. Pharmacy Benefit Management Institute.* Lecture, Orlando, FL.

Granko, R., Morton, C., & Schaafsma, K. (2013). Role of executive coaching in pharmacy management. *American Journal Of Health-System Pharmacy, 70*(21), 1883-1885. doi:10.2146/ajhp130113

Greenfield, R. (2015). *Slacking Off: Can Office Chatrooms Make Us More Productive Time Wasters?*. *Bloomberg*. Retrieved from https://www.bloomberg.com/news/articles/2015-05-21/slacking-off-can-office-chatrooms-makes-us-more-productive-time-wasters-

Gruley, B. (2016). *Is Kratom a Deadly Drug or a Life-Saving Medicine?*. *Bloomberg Businessweek*. Retrieved from https://www.bloomberg.com/news/features/2016-12-12/is-kratom-a-deadly-drug-or-a-life-saving-medicine

Guggenheim, D. (2006). *An Inconvenient Truth*. Hollywood: Paramount Studios.

Gurman, M. (2017). *Apple Wants to Bring Augmented Reality to the Masses. Bloomberg*. Retrieved from https://www.bloomberg.com/news/articles/2017-03-20/apple-s-next-big-thing

Hagemeir, N. & Murawski, M. (2014). An Instrument to Assess Subjective Task Value Beliefs Regarding the Decision to Pursue Postgraduate Training. *American Journal of Pharmaceutical Education, 78*. doi:10.5688/ajpe78111

Hard driving: Uber is facing the biggest crisis in its short history. (2017). *The Economist*. Retrieved from http://www.economist.com/news/business/21719509-can-ride-hailing-giant-stay-fast-lane-uber-facing-biggest-crisis-its-short

Hassler, S. (2016). *STEM Crisis? What About the STS Crisis?*. *IEEE Spectrum*. Retrieved from http://spectrum.ieee. org/at-work/education/stem-crisis-what-about-the-sts-crisis

Hassler, S. (2017). Do we have to build robots that need rights?. *IEEE Spectrum, 54*(3), 6. Retrieved from http:// ieeexplore.ieee.org/stamp/stamp.jsp?tp=&arnumber =7864739&isnumber=7864732

Hatton, R. & Weitzel, K. (2013). Complete-block scheduling for advanced pharmacy practice experiences. *American Journal of Health-System Pharmacy, 70*, 2144-51. doi:10.2146/ajhp130148

Hedgecoe, A. & Martin, P. (2013). The Drugs Don't Work. *Social Studies Of Science, 33*(3), 327-364. doi:10.1177/ 03063127030333002

Herper, M. (2010). *The World's Most Expensive Drugs*. *Forbes*. Retrieved from http://www.forbes. com/2010/02/19/expensive-drugs-cost-business-healthcare-rare-diseases.html

Herper, M. (2016a). *A Biotech's Depression Drug Returns From DEA, Setting Up Test For FDA*. *Forbes*. Retrieved from http://www.forbes.com/sites/matthewherper/ 2016/10/20/biotechs-depression-drug-returns-from-dead-setting-up-test-for-fda/#59a36a5c396b

Herper, M. (2016b). *Billionaire's Former Protege Arrested For Bribing Doctors To Prescribe Fentanyl*.

Forbes. Retrieved from http://www.forbes.com/sites/matthewherper/2016/12/08/billionaires-former-protege-arrested-for-bribing-doctors-to-prescribe-fentanyl/#4f02faa74e64

Heynold, Y. & Rosander, J. (2006). *A new organizational structure for airlines. McKinsey Quarterly.* Retrieved from https://www.mckinseyquarterly.com/A_new_organizational_model_for_airlines_1700

HIE inPractive: Foundation Series. (2013). *Healthcare Information and Management Systems Society.* Retrieved from https://www.himss.org/file/1072106/download?token=lsD8hhMy

Higby, G. (2014). A cornerstone of modern institutional pharmacy practice: Mirror to hospital pharmacy. *American Journal Of Health-System Pharmacy, 71*(22), 1940-1946. doi:10.2146/ajhp140238

Hill, G. (2017). *Wall Street's Outlook on the PBM Industry. Pharmacy Benefit Management Institute.* Lecture, Orlando, FL.

Hossey, M. (2015). *7 Great Works Of Literature (Written While Wasted). Cracked.* Retrieved from http://www.cracked.com/article_22468_7-great-works-literature-written-while-wasted.html

How Target Figured Out A Teen Girl Was Pregnant Before Her Father Did. (2012). *Forbes.* Retrieved from http://www.forbes.com/sites/kashmirhill/2012/02/16/how-target-figured-out-a-teen-girl-was-pregnant-before-her-father-did/

If Computers Wrote Laws: Decisions Handed Down by Data. (2016). *The Economist*. Retrieved from http://worldif.economist.com/article/12133/decisions-handed-down-data

I'll sleep when I'm dead. (2016). *The Economist*. Retrieved from http://www.economist.com/news/international/21690042-working-through-night-probably-shortens-your-life-ill-sleep-when-im-dead

Insulin's Inventor Sold the Patent for $1. Then Drug Companies Got Hold of It.. (2017). *The Other 98%*. Retrieved from https://other98.com/insulins-inventor-sold-patent-1-drug-companies-got-hold/

Internet Law Regulatory and Litigation Matters. (2015). *Journal Of Internet Law, 19*(2), 15-19.

Ishaq Bhatti, M., Awan, H., & Razaq, Z. (2013). The key performance indicators (KPIs) and their impact on overall organizational performance. *Quality & Quantity, 48*(6), 3127-3143. doi:10.1007/s11135-013-9945-y

Jaeger, J. (2009). Boosting control with third-party codes of conduct. *Compliance Week*, (64). 49.

Jain, A. & Kofman, A. (2017). About Faces. *Rhapsody*, 32.

Jarvis, L. (2015a). 2015 was a bountiful year for new drugs. *American Chemical Society: Chemical And Engineering News*, (48), 18. Retrieved from http://cen.acs.org/articles/93/i48/2015-Bountiful-Year-New-Drugs.html

Jarvis, L. (2015b). The Year In New Drugs. *American Chemical Society: Chemical And Engineering News, 93*(5),

11-16. Retrieved from https://cen.acs.org/articles/93/ i5/Year-New-Drugs.html

Johnson, M., Christensen, C., & Kagermann, H. (2008). Re-inventing Your Business Model (cover story). *Harvard Business Review, 86*(12), 50-59.

Johnson, T. & Teeters, J. (2011). Pharmacy residency and the medical training model: Is pharmacy at a tipping point? *American Journal of Health-System Pharmacy, 68*, 1542-9. doi:10.2146/ajhp100483

Jussila, J., Kärkkäinen, H., & Aramo-Immonen, H. (2014). Social media utilization in business-to-business re-lationships of technology industry firms. *Computers in Human Behavior, 30*, 606–613. doi:10.1016/j. chb.2013.07.047

Kachnowski, S. (2017). *Transforming into a Digital Health Era - Are You Ready?. Pharmacy Benefit Management Institute.* Lecture, Orlando, FL.

Kamel, S. & Hussein, M. (2001). The development of e-commerce: The emerging virtual context within Egypt. *Logistics Information Management, 14*(1), 119-126. doi:10.1108/09576050110362555

Karuri, J., Waiganjo, P., Orwa, D., & Manya, A. (2014). DHIS2: The Tool to Improve Health Data Demand and Use in Kenya. *Journal of Health Informatics in Developing Countries*, 8(1), 38-60.

Kassam, R., Kwong, M., & Collins, J. (2013). Clinical Placement Experiences in Long-Term Care Facilities. *BMC*

Medical Education, 13. Retrieved from http://www. biomedcentral.com/1472-6920/13/104

Kirchheimer, S. (2016). *Cut Health Insurance Costs Without Sacrificing Quality of Care. AARP.* Retrieved from http://www.aarp.org/health/health-insurance/ info-2014/cut-health-insurance-costs.html

Kiser, A. (2016). *Someone Didn't Get the Memo. Bloomberg Businessweek.* Retrieved from https:// resourcecenter.businessweek.com/reviews/someone-didnt-get-the-memo

Kiwanuka, A., Kimaro, H., & Senyoni, W. (2015). Analysis of the Acceptance Process of District Health Information Systems (DHIS) for Vertical Health Programmes: A Case Study of TB, HIV/AIDS and Malaria Programmes in Tanzania. *Electronic Journal Of Information Systems In Developing Countries, 70.*

Kondrasuk, J. (2012). The ideal performance appraisal is a format, not a form. *Academy Of Strategic Management Journal, 11*(1), 115-130.

Koyuncu, C. & Lien, D. (2003). E-commerce and consumer's purchasing behavior. *Applied Economics, 35*(6), 721-735.

Kumar, V., Maheshwari, B., & Kumar, U. (2002). Enterprise Resource Planning Systems Adoption Process: A Survey of Canadian Organizations. *International Journal of Production Research, 40*(3), 509-523.

Lalli, F. (2013). Affordable Care Act's 10 Essential Health Benefits. AARP. Retrieved from http://www.aarp.org/

health/health-insurance/info-08-2013/affordable-care-act-health-benefits.html

Landman, A. (2010). *Pfizer and the Big Pharma Felons. PR Watch.* Retrieved from http://www.prwatch.org/spin/2010/11/9645/pfizer-and-big-pharma-felons

Latham, J. (2014). Leadership for quality and innovation: Challenges, theories, and a framework for future research. *Quality Management Journal, 21*(1), 11-15.

Law, J. (2006). *Big pharma* (1st ed.). New York, NY: Carroll & Graf.

Lawrence, E., Culjak, G., & Lawrence, J. (2003). e-Technology v e-Law: Legal challenges to the information society. *Proceedings Of The IADIS International Conference On WWW/Internet,* 971-975.

Lee, A., Son, S., & Kim, K. (2016). Information and communication technology overload and social networking service fatigue: A stress perspective. *Computers in Human Behavior, 55,* 51–61. doi:10.1016/j.chb.2015.08.011

Leotta, A. (2012). *'Law & Order: SVU' Meets 'Fifty Shades of Grey'. The Huffington Post.* Retrieved from http://www.huffingtonpost.com/allison-leotta/law-order-svu-fifty-shades-of-grey_b_1956750.html

Levina, N. & Vaast, E. (2008). Innovating or Doing as Told? Status Differences and Overlapping Boundaries in Offshore Collaboration. *MIS Quarterly, 32*(2), 307-332.

Levitin, D. (2015). *The Organized Mind: Thinking Straight in the Age of Information Overload* (1st ed.). Boston: Dutton.

Lichtblau, L. (1988). Prescribing Within a Range of Reasonableness. *Minnesota Board Of Medical Examiners,* 39-41.

Lin, K. (2011). Simulation and Introductory Pharmacy Practice Experiences. *American Journal of Pharmaceutical Education, 75.* doi:10.5688/ajpe7510209

Livin, A., Hertig, J., & Hultgren, K. (2013). A Call for Standardized Metrics to Assess Health IT Impact on Medication Safety. *Hospital Pharmacy, 48*(10), 801-802. doi:10.1310/hpj4810-801

Llamas, M. (2016). *FDA Says Risks May Outweigh Benefits for Antibiotics Levaquin, Cipro. DrugWatch.* Retrieved from https://www.drugwatch.com/2016/05/16/fda-black-box-warning-for-levaquin-cipro-antibiotic-risk/

Lord, N. (2013). Regulating transnational corporate bribery: Anti-bribery and corruption in the UK and Germany. *Crime, Law & Social Change, 60*(2), 127-145. doi:10.1007/s10611- 013-9445-y

Löscher, P. (2012). The CEO of Siemens On Using a Scandal To Drive Change. *Harvard Business Review, 90*(11), 39-42.

Lucky, R. (2017). *Cozying Up to Complexity. IEEE Explore.* Retrieved from http://ieeexplore.ieee.org/document/7802738/

Luqmani, F. (2014). *Demystifying Cloud Computing.* Lecture.

Manchanda, R. (2016). *The Upstream Effect: What Makes Us Sick?. Quality Talks 2016.* Retrieved from http://www.qualitytalks.org/events/qt-2016/talks/upstream-effect-makes-us-sick/

Mandel, I. & Howson, A. (2015). Causes of Social Change. *Research Starters: Sociology.*

Markman, J. (2016). *Software As A Stock Strategy. Forbes.* Retrieved from http://www.forbes.com/sites/jonmarkman/2016/08/24/software-as-a-stock-strategy/#70f6fb334faf

Mashhadi, S., Hamid, S., Roshan, R., & Fawad, A. (2016). Healthcare in Pakistan – A Systems Perspective. *Pakistan Armed Forces Medical Journal,* (66), 136.

Matavire, R. (2016). Health Information Systems Development: Producing a New Agora in Zimbabwe. *Information Technologies & International Development, 12*(1), 35-50.

McAneny, B. (2016). *Fighting Cancer. Cutting Costs. At the Same Time. Quality Talks 2016.* Retrieved from http://www.qualitytalks.org/events/qt-2016/talks/fighting-cancer-cutting-costs-time/

McCarthy Jr., B. & Weber, L. (2013). Update on factors motivating pharmacy students to pursue residency and fellowship training. *American Journal of Health-System Pharmacy, 70,* 1397-403. doi:10.2146/ajhp120354

Meisner, J. (2009). Customer data breach costs head skyward. *E-Commerce Times, February 3.*

Merchant Warehouse Announces Apple Passbook Acceptance for Genius Customer Engagement Platform. (2012). *MarketWired.* Retrieved from http://www.marketwired.com/press-release/Merchant-Warehouse-

Announces-Apple-Passbook-Acceptance-Genius-Customer-Engagement-1701304.htm

Mieure, K. (2010). A High-Fidelity Simulation Mannequin to Introduce Pharmacy Students to Advanced Cardiovascular Life Support. *American Journal of Pharmaceutical Education, 74.* doi:10.5688/aj740222

Miller, O. (2014). *99 Writers Who Were Alcoholics, Drunks, Addicted To Booze, Etc.. Thought Catalog.* Retrieved from http://thoughtcatalog.com/oliver-miller/2014/03/99-writers-who-were-alcoholics-drunks-addicted-to-booze-etc/

Miller, S. (2017). *Managing a Perfect Storm to Provide the Best in Cost Management and Patient Care. Pharmacy Benefit Management Institute.* Lecture, Orlando, FL.

Mullin, R. (2015). Debate Over The Cost Of Drugs. *American Chemical Society: Chemical And Engineering News,* (48), 20. Retrieved from http://cen.acs.org/articles/93/i48/Debate-Over-Cost-Drugs.html

Murphy, M. (2017). *Melinda Gates on the World's Missing Data About Women. Bloomberg.* Retrieved from https://www.bloomberg.com/news/features/2017-02-14/q-a-melinda-gates-on-the-world-s-missing-data-about-women

Nau, D. (2009). Measuring pharmacy quality. *Journal of the American Pharmacists Association, 49*(2), 154. doi:10.1331/japha.2009.09019

Nawaz, R., Ali Khan, S., & Khan, G. (2015). SWOT Analysis of District Analysis of District Health Information

System in Khyber Pakhtunkhwa. *Gomal Journal Of Medical Sciences, 13*(2), 109-114.

Nyella, E. & Kimaro, H. (2016). HIS Standardization in Developing Countries: Use of Boundary Objects to Enable Multiple Translations. *African Journal Of Information Systems, 8*(1), 64-88.

O'Connor, S. (2013). Interview with John W. Bluford III, FACHE, president and chief executive officer, Truman Medical Centers. *Journal Of Healthcare Management, 58*(6), 389-391.

Onnasch, L., Wickens, C., Li, H., & Manzey, D. (2013). Human Performance Consequences of Stages and Levels of Automation: An Integrated Meta-Analysis. *Human Factors: The Journal Of The Human Factors And Ergonomics Society, 56*(3), 476-488. doi:10.1177/0018720813501549

Osterwalder, A., Pigneur, Y., & Clark, T. (2010). *Business model generation* (1st ed.). Hoboken, N.J.: John Wiley & Sons.

The Other 98%. (2017). *Beautiful Trouble.* Retrieved from http://beautifultrouble.org/partner/the-other-98/

The Other 98% - About. (2010). *Facebook.* Retrieved from https://www.facebook.com/pg/TheOther98/about/?ref=page_internal

Oudshoorn, N. (1993). United We Stand: The Pharmaceutical Industry, Laboratory, and Clinic in the Development of Sex Hormones into Scientific Drugs, 1920-1940. *Science, Technology & Human Values, 18*(1), 5-24. doi:10.1177/016224399301800102

Oxfam says wealth of richest 1% equal to other 99%. (2016). *BBC News.* Retrieved from http://www.bbc.com/news/business-35339475

Palmer, D. (2005). Pop-Ups, Cookies, and Spam: Toward a Deeper Analysis of the Ethical Significance of Internet Marketing Practices. *Journal of Business Ethics, 58*(1-3), 271-280. doi:10.1007/s10551-005-1421-8

Pamfilie, R. & Draghici, M. (2012). The importance of leadership in driving a strategic lean six sigma management. *Procedia - Social And Behavioral Sciences, 58*, 187-196. doi:10.1016/j.sbspro.2012.09.992

Parayitam, S., Desai, K., & Desai, M. (2008). E-Commerce Policies, Customer Privacy and Customer Confidence. *The XIMB Journal Of Management, 5*(2), 45-58.

Patel, J., Sharma, A., West, D., Bates, I., Davies, J., & Abdel-Tawab, R. (2011). An evaluation of using multi-source feedback (MSF) among junior hospital pharmacists. *International Journal Of Pharmacy Practice, 19*(4), 276-280. doi:10.1111/j.2042-7174.2010.00092.x

Patient survey (HCAHPS). (2015). *Medicare Data.* Retrieved from https://data.medicare.gov/Hospital-Compare/Patient-survey-HCAHPS-Hospital/dgck-syfz

Pawloski, P., Cusick, D., & Amborn, L. (2011). Development of clinical pharmacy productivity metrics. *American Journal Of Health-System Pharmacy, 69*(1), 49-54. doi:10.2146/ajhp110126

Pearson v. Chung. (2005). *DC Court Case Records.* Retrieved from https://www.dccourts.gov/cco/maincase.jsf

Peretz, H. & Fried, Y. (2012). National cultures, performance appraisal practices, and organizational absenteeism and turnover: A study across 21 countries. *Journal Of Applied Psychology, 97*(2), 448-459. doi:10.1037/a0026011

Popescu, A. (2017). *These VR Systems Help Treat Veterans Recovering From PTSD. Bloomberg.* Retrieved from https://www.bloomberg.com/news/articles/2017-03-16/these-vr-systems-help-treat-veterans-recovering-from-ptsd

Powell, D., Riezebos, J., & Strandhagen, J. (2013). Lean production and ERP systems in small- and medium-sized enterprises: ERP support for pull production. *International Journal Of Production Research, 51*(2), 395-409. doi:10.1080/00207543.2011.645954

Pretz, K. (2016a). *Yu Yuan's Mission is to Improve Lives Through Virtual Reality. The Institute.* Retrieved from http://theinstitute.ieee.org/members/profiles/yu-yu-ans-mission-is-to-improve-lives-through-virtual-reality

Pretz, K. (2016b). *A New IEEE Initiative Focuses on Augmented Reality, Virtual Reality, and Human Augmentation Technologies. The Institute.* Retrieved from http://theinstitute.ieee.org/technology-topics/consumer-electronics/a-new-ieee-initiative-focuses-on-augmented-reality-virtual-reality-and-human-augmentation-technologies

Purkayastha, D. & Srinivasa Rao, A. (2014). *Corporate Entrepeneurship and Innovation at Google, Inc. The Case*

Centre. Retrieved from http://www.thecasecentre.org/educators/products/view?id=120454

Quelch, J. A. & Rodriguez, M. L. (2013). *GlaxoSmithKline in China (A)*. HBS No. 9-514-049. Boston, MA: Harvard Business School Publishing.

Rafaeli, A. (2013) Emotion in Organizations: Considerations for Family Firms. *Entrepreneurship Research Journal, 3*, 295-299. doi:10.1515/erj-2013-0061

Reconciling e-Commerce and Privacy. (1998). *Businessweek, 10/05/1998*(3598), 194.

Reddy, M., Purao, S., & Kelly, M. (2008). Developing IT Infrastructure for Rural Hospitals: A Case Study of Benefits and Challenges of Hospital-to-Hospital Partnerships. *Journal of the American Medical Informatics Association, 15*(4), 554-558. doi:10.1197/jamia.m2676

Reduce medication errors through following metrics: pharmacy targets workflow issues. (2009). *Drug Formulary Review, 25*(6), 67-69.

Reed, G. (2006). Leadership and Systems Thinking. *Defense AT&L, 35*, 10-13. (AN 20707954)

Rometty, G. (2016). *IBM CEO Ginni Rometty's Letter to the U.S. President-Elect. IBM THINKPolicy*. Retrieved from https://www.ibm.com/blogs/policy/ibm-ceo-ginni-romettys-letter-u-s-president-elect/

Rosenberg, M. (2010). *15 Dirty Big Pharma Tricks That Rip You Off and Risk Your Health for Profit. AlterNet*. Retrieved from http://www.alternet.org/

story/149282/15_dirty_big_pharma_tricks_that_rip_
you_off_and_risk_your_health_for_profit

Rough, S., McDaniel, M., & Rinehart, J. (2010). Effective
use of workload and productivity monitoring tools in
health-system pharmacy, part 1. *American Journal Of
Health-System Pharmacy*, *67*(4), 300-311. doi:10.2146/
ajhp090217.p1

Ru-Chu, S., Chia-Liang, C., Chih-Cheng, T., & Shi-Jer, L.
(2013). Employing Microsoft LIVE@EDU Cloud Platform to Assist in Teaching Chinese Reading for Junior
High School Students. *Turkish Online Journal Of Educational Technology*, *12*(4), 71-74.

Russell, J. (2017). *Pokémon Go has now crossed $1 bil-
lion in revenue. TechCrunch.* Retrieved from https://
techcrunch.com/2017/02/01/report-pokemon-go-
has-now-crossed-1-billion-in-revenue/

Sabar, A. & Lee, S. (2007). *Judge tries suing pants off dry
cleaners. The New York Times.* Retrieved from http://
www.nytimes.com/2007/06/13/us/13pants.html

Sæbø, J., Kossi, E., Titlestad, O., Tohouri, R., & Braa, J.
(2011). Comparing strategies to integrate health information systems following a data warehouse approach
in four countries. *Information Technology For Development*, *17*(1), 42-60.

Sampson, J. & Makela, J. (2014). Ethical issues associated with information and communication technology
in counseling and guidance. *International Journal of*

Educational and Vocational Guidance, 14(1), 135-148. doi:10.1007/s10775-013-9258-7

Satya Nadella. (2017). *Forbes.* Retrieved from https://www.forbes.com/profile/satya-nadella/?list=powerful-people

Satya Nadella email to employees on first day as CEO. (2016). *Microsoft News.* Retrieved from http://news.microsoft.com/2014/02/04/satya-nadella-email-to-employees-on-first-day-as-ceo/

Scahill, S. (2008). *Improving community pharmacy services by studying organizational theory. Southern Med Review, 1*(1), 17-20.

Schaefer, K. (2016). *Stop Monday From Ruining Your Sunday. Bloomberg.com.* Retrieved from https://www.bloomberg.com/news/articles/2016-10-14/stop-monday-from-ruining-your-sunday

Scott, S. & Einstein, W. (2001). Strategic performance appraisal in team-based organizations: One size does not fit all. *Academy Of Management Executive, 15*(2), 107-116. doi:10.5465/ame.2001.4614990

Seabury, S. (2012). Jury verdicts, settlement behavior and expected trial outcomes. *International Review of Law and Economics, 33.* Retrieved from http://www.sciencedirect.com/science/journal/01448188/33?sdc=1

Security Terms Unlocked. (2017). *CyberTrend.* Retrieved from https://www.cybertrend.com/article/23891/security-terms-unlocked

Seybert, A. (2007). Simulation-Based Learning to Teach Blood Pressure Assessment to Doctor of Pharmacy Students. *American Journal of Pharmaceutical Education, 71*. doi:10.5688/aj710348

Sharma, G. & Lijuan, W. (2014). Ethical perspectives on e-commerce: an empirical investigation. *Internet Research, 24*(4), 414-435. doi:10.1108/intr-07-2013-0162

Shobert, B. & DeNoble, D. (2013). Compliance After China's Healthcare Bribery Scandals. *China Business Review, 11*.

Shortliffe, E. & Cimino, J. (2013). *Biomedical Informatics: Computer Applications in Health Care and Biomedicine* (4th ed.). London: Springer.

Silberman, S. (2009). *Placebos Are Getting More Effective. Drugmakers Are Desperate to Know Why. WIRED.* Retrieved from https://www.wired.com/2009/08/ff-placebo-effect/

Smith, K. (2015). Transgender employees: The new protected category?. *New York Employment Law, 10*(2), 6.

Stoughton, J., Thompson, L., & Meade, A. (2013). Big five personality traits reflected in job applicants' social media postings. *Cyberpsychology, Behavior, And Social Networking, 16*(11), 800-805. doi:10.1089/cyber.2012.0163

Sullivan, A. (2007). *Judge persists in suing the pants off dry cleaners; Washington D.C. bencher appeals to pursue $54 million lawsuit. The Vancouver Sun.*

Sung, J. (2016). *Protecting Affordable Health Insurance Premiums for Older Adults. AARP.* Retrieved from http://blog.aarp.org/2016/12/29/protecting-afford-able-health-insurance-premiums-for-older-adults/

Tennissen, M. (2007). *Local case recalls the 1994 hot coffee 'Mc Lawsuit.' Southeast Texas Record.* Retrieved from www.lexisnexis.com/hottopics/lnacademic

Territo, J. (2016). *Performance Reporting: Easing Your Grief. Quality Talks 2016.* Retrieved from http://www.qualitytalks.org/events/qt-2016/talks/performance-reporting-easing-grief/

Thayer, A. (2015). Leading Drugs Under Fire In 2015. *American Chemical Society: Chemical And Engineering News, 93*(48), 19. Retrieved from https://cen.acs.org/articles/93/i48/Leading-Drugs-Under-Fire-2015.html

Thayer, A. (2017). AbbVie's Humira held onto top spot despite biosimilar threat. *American Chemical Society: Chemical And Engineering News.* Retrieved from http://yearinreview.cenmag.org/abbvies-humira-held-onto-top-spot-despite-biosimilar- threat/

Tim Cook. (2017). *Forbes.* Retrieved from https://www.forbes.com/profile/tim-cook/?list=powerful-people

Tiwari, V., Kumar, K., Raj, S., & Kulkarni, P. (2016). Standards, Frameworks and Practices in Health Management Information and Evaluation Systems (HMIES) in Australia and India: Lessons for Future Transition in India?. *Journal Of Health Management, 18*(1), 70- 83.

Tofil, N. (2010). Use of Simulation to Enhance Learning in a Pediatric Elective. *American Journal of Pharmaceutical Education, 74.* doi:0.5688/aj740221

Tuckson, R. (2016). *Telehealth Is Revolutionizing Care Delivery: Can It Change the Value Definition?. Quality Talks 2016.* Retrieved from http://www.qualitytalks.org/events/qt-2016/talks/telehealth-revolutionizing-care-delivery-can-change-value-definition/

U.S. Department of Health and Human Services (HHS), Office of the Surgeon General, *Facing Addiction in America: The Surgeon General's Report on Alcohol, Drugs, and Health.* Washington, DC: Health and Human Services, November 2016.

Understanding Medicare, Getting Started. (2016). *AARP.* Retrieved from http://www.aarp.org/health/medicare-insurance/info-01-2011/understanding_medicare_a_boomers_guide.html

Vardi, N. (2016). *Moderna's Mysterious Medicines. Forbes.* Retrieved from http://www.forbes.com/sites/nathanvardi/2016/12/14/modernas-mysterious-medicines/#762336ec730e

Visibility to bring full ERP to Apple iPad device. (2010). *Tendersinfo News.*

Vivekananda-Schmidt, P., MacKillop, L., Crossley, J., & Wade, W. (2013). Do assessor comments on a multi-source feedback instrument provide learner-centred feedback?. *Medical Education, 47*(11), 1080-1088. doi:10.1111/medu.12249

Volkow, N. (2016). *Treating Addiction Within the Health Care System. Quality Talks 2016.* Retrieved from http://www.qualitytalks.org/events/qt-2016/talks/treating-addiction-within-health-care-system/

Walters, N. (2016). *CEO Ginni Rometty: people from Facebook come to IBM to "have an impact on serious things". TheStreet.* Retrieved from https://www.thestreet.com/story/13675433/2/ceo-ginni-rometty-tells-bloomberg-businessweek-how-ibm-plans-to-compete-with-google.html

We Are the 99 Percent. (2017). *We Are The 99 Percent.* Retrieved from http://wearethe99percent.tumblr.com/Introduction

Webb, A. (2017). *Sweetening the Deal. Bloomberg Businessweek.*

Webfortis and Microsoft Announce Apple Watch App for Dynamics CRM and Parature. (2015). *Global Newswire.* Retrieved from https://globenewswire.com/news-release/2015/07/12/751329/0/en/Webfortis-and-Microsoft-Announce-Apple-Watch-App-for-Dynamics-CRM-and-Parature.html

Weinberg, N. & Langreth, R. (2017). *Drug Costs Too High? Fire the Middleman. Bloomberg.* Retrieved from https://www.bloomberg.com/news/articles/2017-03-03/drug-costs-too-high-fire-the-middleman

What is value? definition and meaning. (2017). *Business Dictionary.* Retrieved from http://www.businessdictionary.com/definition/value.html

What Satya Nadella did at Microsoft. (2017). *The Economist.* Retrieved from http://www.economist.com/news/business/21718916-worlds-biggest-software-firm-has-transformed-its-culture-better-getting-cloud

White, S. (2005). Will there be a pharmacy leadership crisis? An ASHP foundation scholar-in-residence report. *American Journal of Health-System Pharmacy, 62*(8), 845-855.

White, S. (2006). Leadership: Successful alchemy. *American Journal Of Health-System Pharmacy, 63*(16), 1497-1503. doi:10.2146/ajhp060263

Williams, L. & Wilkins. (2016). Costs of US prescription opioid epidemic estimated at $78.5 billion. *ScienceDaily.* doi:10.1097/MLR.0000000000000625

Williamson, L., Kaasbøll, J., Braa, J., & Sun, V. (2008). South-South Collaboration: Adapting Information Systems Integration Strategies in Namibia. *IST-Africa 2008 Conference Proceedings.* Paul Cunningham and Miriam Cunningham (Eds).

Wu, K., Yang, L., & Chiang, I. (2012). Leadership and six sigma project success: The role of member cohesiveness and resource management. *Production Planning & Control, 23*(9), 707-717. doi:10.1080/09537287.2011.586650

Yeung, L., Cheng, K., Fong, C., Lee, W., & Tong, K. (2014). Evaluation of the Microsoft Kinect as a clinical assessment tool of body sway. *Gait & Posture, 40*(4), 532-538. doi:10.1016/j.gaitpost.2014.06.012

Yohay, P. (1977). DC Consumer Protection Procedures Act. *Catholic University Law Review, 27*, 642-652.

Yonce, C. (2015). How Your Favorite Companies and Causes Use BI to Succeed. *Business Intelligence Journal*, 38-41.

Young, S., Vos, S., Cantrell, M., & Shaw, R. (2014) Factors Associated With Students' Perception of Preceptor Excellence. *American Journal of Pharmaceutical Education, 78*. doi:10.5688/ajpe78353

Zaharia, G., Zaharia, C., Tudorescu, N., & Zaharia, I. (2010). Online Crime and the Regulation of Business on the Internet. *Economics, Management & Financial Markets, 5*(4), 238-243.

Zillman, C. (2017). *At Davos, IBM CEO Ginni Rometty Downplays Fears of a Robot Takeover. Fortune*. Retrieved from http://fortune.com/2017/01/18/ibm-ceo-ginni-rometty-ai-davos/

Zimmer, C. (2012). *Law & Order SVU 'Twenty-Five Acts' Recap & Review. All Things Law and Order*. Retrieved from https://allthingslawandorder.blogspot.com/2012/10/law-order-svu-twenty-five-acts-recap.html?m=1

Appendix C: Recommended Reading

Anderson, K. (2017). *Retire on Real Estate: Building Rental Income for a Safe and Secure Retirement* (1st ed.). New York: American Management Association.

Arbesman, S. (2012). *The Half-Life of Facts: Why Everything We Know has an Expiration Date* (1st ed.). New York: Penguin Group.

DeCleene, J. (2009). *Medical Adventures: Inspired by a True Story* (1st ed.). Bloomington: AuthorHouse.

Gladwell, M. (2002). *The Tipping Point.* New York: Back Bay Books.

Gladwell, M. (2009). *Outliers: The Story of Success.* New York: Back Bay Books.

Guggenheim, D. (2006). *An Inconvenient Truth.* Hollywood: Paramount Studios.

Law, J. (2006). *Big Pharma: Exposing the Global Healthcare Agenda* (1st ed.). New York: Carroll & Graf.

Martin, J. (2007). *The Meaning of the 21st Century: A Vital Blueprint for Ensuring Our Future* (1st ed.). New York: Riverhead Trade.

Noah, T. (2016). *Born a Crime: Stories from a South African Childhood* (1st ed.). New York: Random House.

Osterwalder, A., Pigneur, Y., & Clark, T. (2013). *Business Model Generation: A Handbook for Visionaries, Game Changers, and Challengers* (1st ed.). Hoboken: John Wiley & Sons.

Tyson, N. (2017). *Astrophysics for People in a Hurry* (1st ed.). New York: Norton, W. W. & Company, Inc.

About the Author

Justin DeCleene MBA, MIS, CPhT started with humble beginnings in Green Bay, WI. In 2008, he wrote his first book *Medical Adventures: Inspired by a True Story*. Upon completing high school in three years, he moved to Baltimore, MD to start his college career. After earning his Bachelors of Science in Chemistry, he took a 180° turn in his career path and started working on his Master's in Business Administration which led him to pursue his Master's in Information Systems. Justin still resides in Baltimore and has used his expertise in healthcare, business, and technology to successfully manage multiple projects in a fast-paced environment. He has effectuated change within an organization across multiple departments and provided training to foster that change. He has critiqued information systems and proposed enhancements to better align with the organization's requirements. With this book, Justin hopes to inspire the next generation to utilize bodies of information to potentiate positive change across the globe.